9.14.78

Eat OK — Feel OK!

Food Facts and Your Health

By the Same Authors:

— Elizabeth M. Whelan and Fredrick J. Stare
Panic in the Pantry: Food Facts, Fads and Fallacies   *1975*
     (Trans. into Japanese, 1976, and into French, 1977)

— Fredrick J. Stare
Living Nutrition (2nd Edition)   1977
Nutrition for Good Health   1974
Eating for Good Health   1964

— Elizabeth M. Whelan
Preventing Cancer: What You Can Do
     to Cut Your Risks By Up to 50%   1978
Boy or Girl?   1977
A Baby? . . . Maybe   1975
Making Sense Out of Sex   1975
Sex and Sensibility   1974

Eat OK — Feel OK!

Food Facts and Your Health

By

FREDRICK J. STARE, M.D., Ph.D.
Professor of Nutrition at the
Harvard School of Public Health

and

ELIZABETH M. WHELAN, M.P.H., Sc.D.
Executive Director of the American
Council on Science and Health

THE CHRISTOPHER PUBLISHING HOUSE
NORTH QUINCY, MASSACHUSETTS

PRINTED IN
THE UNITED STATES OF AMERICA

Acknowledgments

We'd like to thank those individuals who were particularly helpful in the preparation of this book and those who participated over the last few years in the writing of the syndicated column "Food and Your Health."

We are especially indebted to Cynthia Ford, M.S., Marie Alexander, M.S., Johanna Dwyer, D.S., Madge Myers, M.S., Patricia S. Remmell, M.S., Mary B. McCann, M.D., Joyce Moody, M.Ed., and George Kerr, M.D. for their work on "Food and Your Health," and to Marilyn King Bartle and June Miller for typing the various drafts of this manuscript.

Contents

Introduction

This book would probably have caught your eye quicker if it had been entitled *"The Martini and Olive Diet"* or *"The Revolutionary Way to Good Health Through the Newly Discovered Vitamin Q-8"* or even *"Other Things to Do in Bed to Keep Slim—Eat Crackers."* However, we decided that *Eat OK—Feel OK!* best fits the time and subject matter. In short, we hope that you will read this book and improve your health by eating for good health.

If you look around your local bookstore you'll see dozens of so-called "health and diet guides" which promise to solve your on-going problem of living beyond your seams while at the same time leave you glowing with natural, organically-derived vitality. Usually these books have three things in common: they boast of spectacular new findings which have rocked the nutritional foundations of the world, and they predict instantaneous results. In those two ways they are very appealing. After all, we live in an impatient world where things change very fast, and if we hear of a shortcut to anything, including improved health, we're interested in finding out more. But the third thing these books usually have in common is the clinker: they generally are based on little or no scientific fact, they don't work and they may possibly be harmful to your health.

Regardless of how you interpret the book's main title, *Eat OK—Feel OK!* doesn't have any gimmicks, and it does have many tips on how to ensure that you and your family stay healthy through sensible eating. It doesn't have any "revolutionary" new formulas for "girth control." But it does present scientifically based no-nonsense steps you can take if you have some fat that does not fit.

It doesn't tell you that you are poisoning yourself to death by eating food additives and pesticides, and it does not berate the food industry, Food and Drug Administration and the local butcher for serving us unfit food. Instead, it emphasizes that we do have good foods in this country—as good as, if not better than, in any country in the world.   The Department of Agriculture, Food and Drug Administration, Public Health Service, National Academy of Sciences, to say nothing of the excellent laboratories of many of the food and chemical companies—and let's not forget our universities— have done and are doing an outstanding job to give us good, safe food—and plenty of it. Of course this is not the currently popular position to take. It's much easier and, as I pointed out above, saleable to take the poisons-in-your-food stance and offer some "natural organic" alternatives to allegedly safer—and certainly more expensive—eating.

In the pages that follow, you'll find a practical overview of the field of nutrition, that is, the science of food and its relation to health.   We begin with the basics—the building blocks of good nutrition, protein, carbohydrates, fats, vitamins, minerals and water. Yes, most of our foods have more water than anything else—milk has more than 90 percent water and so do most fruits and vegetables; meats have 65-75 percent water and so does your body. And some drinking waters are good sources of minerals, including the essential mineral fluoride.   If you take the time to understand how all of the nutrients our body needs function together you'll be better prepared to meet the challenges of your faddist friends who recommend "lots of this vitamin, no carbohydrates and supplements of Aunt Matilda's Homemade Kelp" or someone's bone meal.

With these basics set forth, we discuss how to apply the nutritional premises of varied well-balanced meals to everyday living and take a long, hard (and critical) look at the current American fascination with the "eat, drink and supplement" philosophy. Since eating in our modern world requires some degree of nutritional sophistication, we focus a few chapters on our current forms of food processing, food safety, the use of food additives and preservatives, new "imitation" foods, and what we know right now about the relationship of food and disease. And because each age— infancy, childhood, teen-age, pregnancy, lactation and the golden years—have their own individual nutritional requirements, and since many of us have unique dietary formulas we have to follow, you'll find a full chapter on "Special Needs."

And what would a food book be without some extensive comments about weight control?   Chapter seven will give you some clues about how to cope with (or even better, *prevent*) the bulging that comes from overindulging and will offer some specific comments about the widely publicized fad diets which, if you are serious about keeping your weight down, you should carefully avoid.

Much of the commentary in this book is based on my twice-weekly syndicated newspaper column "Food and Your Health," that I have managed, with the help of my associates, to get out for the last twenty-five years. "Food and Your Health" has become quite popular and has given me the opportunity to keep up-to-date on questions and concerns of eaters in the United States and Canada. "Fan mail" averages several hundred letters a week. The numbers go up when we step on the toes of food faddists, die-hard anti-fluoridationists or those of the poisons-in-your-pantry advocates. Generally these are the same toes.

In the appendices of this book you'll find some of the most frequently asked questions (arranged by topic) which I've answered in that column over the years and an example of some of the quizzes I've tried out on my newspaper column readers. You should try them too to determine your nutritional IQ. Why not try it both before and after you read the book!

We hope these pages will prove useful to you. What we have written, to the best of our knowledge, represents sense on nutrition, not nonsense. Balanced, nutritious eating is not a fad. It is not something you do for two weeks or two months and then forget about. Eating for good health is a lifetime matter. And what better time to start than right now?

Fredrick J. Stare, M.D.
Professor of Nutrition
Harvard School of Public Health
Boston, Massachusetts

Chapter One
Beware of Nutritional Hogwash!

Will gullible eaters swallow anything?

One begins to think so after surveying some of the nutritional advice which currently surrounds us—molecular psychiatry, megavitamins, "one hundred percent natural—no artificial anything" foods, and the so-called "fat burning" diet regimens which claim to have the same effect on your corpulence as a sudden rise in temperature has on Frosty the Snowperson.

And of course there are the standard miracle foods which assure the perpetual glow of health. Dried alfalfa. Lecithin. Blackstrap Molasses. Honey. Vinegar. Wheat germ. In this category, wheat germ probably holds the top honors. Today some people are eating so much wheat germ they are beginning to sway in the breeze.

Despite the abundance of a variety of attractive, inexpensive nutritious foods, some eaters today insist on limiting their diet to a small number of specialty items, some of which don't sound very appetizing, many of which have questionable nutritional value, and all of which put an unnecessary strain on the pocketbook. Can you imagine enjoying a tall glass of chilled seawater? Or how about some nice, natural, unpasteurized milk, complete with its risk of undulant fever and tuberculosis? And of course there are hot dogs sold in some parts of health-food-land without benefit of the preservatives that prevent botulism.

Nutritional nonsense and health hazards surround us. Many of those who should be well informed about what they should and should not eat are abandoning common sense in favor of a fad diet. Probably the most outrageous—and admittedly extreme—"strange eating story" was reported in a 1968 issue of the journal *Nutrition Today*. It seems that a gentleman from Darwin, Australia devised his own "mechanical diet," making a bet with a friend that he could eat a standard-sized automobile over the course of four years. Evidently he wished to take his iron au naturel. Follow-up reports did not indicate if this individual actually did eat the entire car and, if he did, whether he developed a spare tire.

What's going on? Why are so many people rejecting the science of nutrition in favor of food faddism? Why are some eaters so willing— indeed eager—to accept the counsel of a radio announcer, writers with no background in the area of food science, alarmists who appear to have made a career out of stirring up consumer concerns, and activists who are strong on activism but weak on nutrition? Why are people turning to "quick loss diets" when they really know that there is just one thing a wishful shrinker should eat—less?

The answers to these questions are complex, but in pondering them it's useful to step back for a moment and put the question in perspective. It's easy initially to assume that food faddism and experimentation with "magic foods" and "revolutionary new diets" are unique to our time. They are not. Ever since the time of Adam, people have had complaints about their food. And some of our earliest medical records document that the concern about excess weight (particularly among affluent people) is hardly a novel one.

Ancient Hogwash

The food nonsense which was fed to the public in earlier years was more understandable. It is, after all, only relatively recent in our history that we began to understand what the basis of good nutrition was. In earlier centuries, for instance, medical researchers experimented with "food cures" and various eating styles and, if they lived to tell about it, drew spectacular conclusions.

Pliny recommended cucumbers for "hot stomachs and hot livers." Egyptians fed sick children skinned mice. In 1689 a prominent Italian physician identified walnut juice as the key to perfect nutrition, a source of long life and health. In 1715 an English surgeon claimed that sugar alone could provide the basis for good nutrition, good disposition and a cure for all wounds. Another eighteenth-century doctor recommended vinegar as the cure for yellow fever. And in the late nineteenth century a German physician, Dr. L. Schenck, advocated the elimination of all starch and sugar from the diet of a pregnant woman who hoped for a son. Of course, since girls were made of sugar and spice, the recipe was reversed if a daughter was desired.

Garlic is a food which has had good and bad reviews. While the ancients claimed that it was an excellent food to both clean out arteries and open obstructions, and others recommended the use of garlic suppositories for cleansing the blood and intestines, still others condemned the herb as the primary underlying cause of "sexual excess." Perhaps next year garlic will be "in" again, possibly even replacing vitamin E as the cure-all for sexual inadequacy!

These early counselors just didn't have the science of nutrition to turn to. They were on their own. Each tried his own formula. Obviously some of these "tips for health" were harmless as well as ineffective. Some, however, including the elimination of basic nutrients from the diet of a pregnant woman posed a real threat to her and her unborn child.

Other such experiments quickly proved fatal. For instance, the story of William Starr, M.D., is an interesting one to consider. This young physician, writing in a diary in 1770, described himself as being twenty-nine years old, six feet tall with red hair and "stoutly made but not corpulent." Dr. Starr had an interest in good nutrition and healthy living (and so does Dr. Stare!), and on the advice of an acquaintance decided to modify his diet. The acquaintance was Benjamin Franklin.

Dr. Starr's diary reports that "Dr. B. Franklin of Philadelphia informed me that he himself when a journeyman printer had lived a fortnight on bread and water at the rate of ten pounds of bread a week and found himself stout and hearty on this diet." Noting that poor people often didn't eat animal food and seemed to be healthy, Dr. Starr decided to limit himself to twenty to thirty-eight ounces of bread daily with water. After a few weeks of this less than appealing and certainly unnourishing menu, he treated himself to a bit of sugar too. Within weeks his diary account began to report failing health: "I now perceive small ulcers on the inside of my cheeks, particularly near a bad tooth; the gums of the upper jaw of the same side were swelled and red and bled when pressed with the finger."

But Dr. Starr persevered. Bread, water, sugar and on special occasions some olive oil. He died at the age of thirty, a victim of self-inflicted scurvy.

But, you say, something like that could never happen today. We're too nutritionally sophisticated. Unfortunately—tragically—a variation of Dr. Starr's experiment is reflected in the cases of confirmed Zen Macrobiotic eaters who insist on limiting food intake to brown rice to achieve an "ideal" balance of "yin and yang." Strict adherence to this diet in recent years has posed serious and sometimes lethal threats: the well-publicized starvation death of twenty-four-year-old Mrs. Beth Ann Simon was a grim reminder of the consequences of extreme food faddism and self-prescribed experiments.

The Revolutionary, New 1863 Diet!

Do you think our diet craze is something new? Certainly it's more significant now than ever before, but it is definitely not new. Diet advice has flourished for years, that is, it has among those individuals who had enough food to eat in the first place. We'll consider just two random examples.

Socrates was concerned about his weight. His solution? He advised dancing before breakfast as a means of keeping slim. And he offered us the following philosophy to keep in mind as we approach the dinner table, "Bad men live that they may eat and drink, whereas good men eat and drink so that they may live."

But let's jump ahead closer to modern time for a second example. In 1863, an English surgeon named William Harvey (not to be confused with another Dr. William Harvey who in times past described the mechanisms of blood circulation) devised a diet for his corpulent patients. He specifically forbade sweet and starchy foods while permitting as much meat as they cared to eat. Indeed, one of his portly patients, William Banting, attested to the efficacy of the Harvey diet in *A Letter on Corpulence Addressed to the Public* (1863). He thought the diet was great; he lost some weight—if only temporarily.

Does this low-carbohydrate/high-protein diet sound familiar to you? You'll find it in various forms at your local bookstore, most likely with a title which includes the term "revolutionary." As we'll point out in our later discussion of weight control, the 1863 Harvey diet—complete with its inherent health problems—cyclically appears on book lists under new eye-catching titles. Gullible readers then buy them and eagerly devour a few hundred pages of old-fashioned nonsense.

Why All the Fuss About Food Now?

It doesn't seem to make sense. We've got the facts about well-balanced human nutrition, and we know the way to safe, long-term weight control. There is no mystery any more.

Why do we still see books around by authors such as Dr. Melvin Page (a dentist) who claims that milk drinking is unnatural and the underlying cause of colds, sinusitis, colitis and cancer? Near that you might see the work of another pseudo-nutritionist, the late Jerome Rodale, who in his book *My Own Technique of Eating for Health* agrees with Page, presenting as his Number One Natural Guideline "no milk." And we're back to the question "why" again.

As we've mentioned, concerns about food and dieting have always been with us. Food philosophies have a very emotional base, and people tend to defend them irrationally, usually without benefit of facts. If you have ever tried to argue a point with a confirmed food faddist, you understand the intensity of the feelings involved. But today there's more than that underlying aberrations in eating behavior. The "normal" amount of food concern and experimentation is complicated by two factors.

First, American consumers—possibly you among them—are more puzzled than ever before about "those chemicals" in food. And your questions and concerns are fully understandable.

Do you remember in 1969 when the artificial sweetener cyclamate was removed from the market? Right about that time people began to cross-examine food labels, notice some unpronounceable chemical names and began to feel uneasy. When, in the early 1970s, newspapers carried numerous stories about investigations into the safety of other food additives (coloring agents, the flavor enhancer MSG, the nitrates and nitrites in bacon, for instance) more and more stomachs began to churn. Concerns intensified with the banning of red dye # 2 — and the proposed banning of saccharin. At the same time new food substitutes were being introduced and labels more frequently carried the mysterious words "enriched" or "fortified."

What a perfect setting for a "natural" foods movement to thrive! In the background was a concern which is on the minds of all of us: the threat of cancer and other dread diseases and our questions about what causes them. Well, why not blame food additives and "unnatural eating"!

Of course there is no proof that our unsolved diseases and ad-

additives are linked, except perhaps for the evidence we have that certain additives we'll discuss in later chapters may be influential in *reducing* risks of, for instance, stomach cancer. Nor is there even a shred of evidence that additives, such as cyclamate, which were called into question and/or banned, ever posed any threat to human health. But the recipe for a food fad does not call for facts. Suspicion and fear—mixed liberally with undocumented claims about miracle foods—are the only ingredients necessary. Mother Nature and her early associates can then cash in on the results.

Second, we're living in an age of "calorie anxiety." We have thin standards of beauty and health—and fat standards of living. We want it both ways: our 3,000 Calories a day *and* our size-six dress or thirty-two-inch-waist trousers. With this kind of conflict, no wonder Americans are an easy target for "quick-weight-loss" diets. These regimens are appealing because they seem to offer something for nothing, except, of course, the nonrefundable fee for the author's book. (Actually what they are offering is "nothing" for "something.") Combining a fervent desire to lose weight with a negligible amount of willpower, you have the exact mold the diet-fad recipes call for.

But here you are, still wondering about the food you're now eating and the diet you might go on. Should you continue to be concerned with the food you buy, eyeing it suspiciously to figure out if it is "overprocessed" and filled with poisons? Should you try your great aunt's advice on including health-food store supplements in your diet? Or the advice of your well-meaning neighbor who is on an ecology jag but is not quite sure what ecology is? Should you give the fad diets a try because "Well, maybe there's something to them"? No. No. No. And No.

But there is something you can do. You can get the facts, by far the best ammunition against food and diet faddism and most definitely your answer to better eating and healthier living. So read on!

Chapter Two
What's There to Eat?

KNOW THY NUTRIENTS!

Well, what can we eat? The answer to that is simple: a variety of good, wholesome, health-promoting food, just the very kind you find in your friendly local supermarket!

There is no one "perfect food." The human body needs a variety of materials to function properly. You thought milk was the perfect food, even though it is mostly water? Well, actually, it is the one food that comes close to earning that title because it provides more nutritive value per serving than any other naturally existing food. It's a marvelous (and delicious!) part of our diet, but it can't single-handedly keep us going. We've all heard about various "milk diets" (at the end of it your weight is measured in quarts and pints!), but limiting yourself to one food, even one as good as milk, is nutritionally unsound.

What are the nutrients we need? You probably studied many of them in high school and could recite the names of some and the names of the diseases which occurred when you didn't have enough of one or the other. You certainly learned that iron is necessary for good red blood (and milk is essentially devoid of iron!). But to ensure that you are well prepared to wage the war against food faddism, it's worthwhile reviewing the basics of nutrition which revolve around six essentials of life: protein, carbohydrates, fats, vitamins, minerals and water.

The purpose of this review is merely to give you an introduction to nutritional basics. It will be in chapter three that we'll focus more closely on the application of these facts to the everyday meal planning at your household. Let's look first at protein.

Protein

If you were taking a popularity poll on the various essential nutrients, protein would probably come out far ahead of the rest. It has a good image. What do you think of when you hear the word protein? Strength. Vitality. Health. All those are true, but to keep things in perspective, remember that protein is just one of the ingredients in the magic recipe for good health.

If you want the scientific definition, proteins are unique organic compounds containing nitrogen. They are made of amino acids, some twenty-two and all "nasty old chemicals." After water, and possibly fat, protein is the most plentiful substance in the body. It occurs in all body tissues and fluids. Indeed its name gives a clue to its importance: it is derived from the Greek word meaning "holding first place."

So what has protein done for us lately? Many things, actually, most of which we take for granted: for instance, like keeping our blood cells healthy, ensuring that we have antibodies to fight disease, and producing hormones and enzymes to regulate our body cells. Check the "what they do" section of the chart on pages 41-46, and be grateful for protein. In this country where meat and meat products, poultry, fish, legumes, milk and cereals are plentiful, unless you go on some weird type of protein-low diet, you'll have little trouble meeting your protein needs. Unfortunately, in developing countries, the situation is often very different.

You should be aware that there are two types of proteins in your foods. As mentioned, all proteins are made of small units called amino acids. Eight of the known twenty-two amino acids are essential parts of the human diet. They cannot be built by our bodies, as can the other amino acids. We must take them in our food. When a protein has all of the eight essential amino acids, as well as most of the others, it is called a *complete protein*. *Incomplete proteins*, which are those lacking in one or more of the eight essential amino acids, include the proteins of wheat, corn, rice, and other cereal-like products, vegetables such as soybeans, navy beans, lentils, lima and pinto beans, potatoes, peas and peanut butter. In terms of world nutrition, cereals provide more protein than all foods combined.

This distinction between the types of protein doesn't mean that you should have a grudge against your breakfast cereal and dinner vegetables. But you should keep in mind that meeting your protein needs means mixing your protein sources such as cereal and milk or bread and cheese. This can be a problem for an individual who is a strict vegetarian and avoids even animal products such as cheese, eggs and milk. But we'll get into that topic in chapter six.

Carbohydrates

In that nutrient popularity poll, carbohydrates, that is, the essential starches, sugars and cellulose, probably wouldn't fare very well. Particularly in recent years, carbohydrates have had a bad press. Everyone is talking about avoiding them! The comedian Sam Levenson, for instance, in describing one of his many attempts at dieting wrote of his woes in the battle against carbohydrates and his concern that the starch would sneak unnoticed from the tablecloth and his shirts into his digestive system. And another carbohydrate, sugar, has been blamed for everything from tooth decay and diabetes to coronary heart disease.

As we'll point out later, the charges against various carbohydrates are not backed up by facts. (Starches play an important role in human nutrition, and sugar is not a cause of either diabetes or heart disease and only causes problems with regard to tooth decay when it is taken between meals, particularly in sticky snack foods. Sugar taken with meals is no more responsible for tooth decay than any other food in the human diet.) Food and the bacteria normally present in the mouth are the causes of tooth decay. The only sure way to prevent tooth decay completely is to never let food come in contact with your teeth. And drinking fluoridated water from infancy throughout life will reduce tooth decay by 60 to 70 percent, regardless of what you eat! But still carbohydrates are given bad reviews.

Together with fats, starches and sugars supply the body with relatively inexpensive sources of energy. Additionally, another carbohydrate, cellulose (currently referred to as fiber) plays an important part in providing bulk in the intestinal tract, encouraging the motility of foods through the digestive system. (Cellulose and all other types of fiber are not digested and are not important sources of energy for humans.)

Furthermore, carbohydrates also supply the body with important building materials. If you do not take in enough carbohydrate (or fat, see the next section) your body will be forced to deplete protein supplies as a source of energy. You can't eat your cake and also save it; that is, use protein for energy and also have it to make enzymes and hormones.

So we do need carbohydrates, and don't let anyone tell you otherwise! You find them in such foods as wheat, corn, rice, oats, and food made from these sources, for instance, spaghetti, macaroni, breakfast cereals, noodles and breads. Other sources of carbohydrates include potatoes, sweet potatoes, oats, vegetables such as peas, dried beans, peanuts and soybeans.

How much carbohydrate do we need? The answer to that question is that while carbohydrates are essential for a well-balanced diet, the individual need can vary. In our country, for instance, a typical diet of 2,500 Calories would contain about 280 grams of carbohydrates (about ten ounces), but this amount could be decreased or increased by half and still one could have a well-balanced diet if the food providing the rest of the calories were properly selected.

In general, 40-60 percent of total calories in our typical diet are provided by carbohydrates, usually divided into one-third sugar and two-thirds starch. Don't be afraid of carbohydrates! Cut down on them if you like, but certainly don't eliminate them—even for the short duration of a fad diet. And if you are interested in taking off some weight, cut down on all sources of calories and increase the use of calories, that is, be more active physically—walk, run, play "huffing and puffing" games, even exercise!

Fats

For those not trained in science, fat is a dirty word. Even worse than carbohydrates. You might think of fat people, animal fats, cooking fats and every food on the list of those you like which also happens to be on the list excluded from your low calorie diet.

But again we need fats, although not as many of them as most of us typically now consume. First, fats play the important role of contributing palatability to our food and giving us a feeling of being satisfied—satiety value. Pastries and other baked products, for instance, are tender and delicious because they have fat. Second, fats carry the fat-soluble vitamins A, D and E and are essential parts of the structure of the cells which make up body tissues. There is another fat-soluble vitamin—K, but it is skimpy in all foods. We get it more from the bacteria that normally inhabit our lower intestine and make it for us. Third, our body fats protect vital organs by providing cushions around them, and they help insulate the body and conserve body heat.

The problem, of course, is when the fats around our middle and elsewhere become too plentiful. The average American daily calorie intake consists of some 40-50 percent fat. Most nutritionists believe that is too much. We'd probably all be better off if we could keep our fat intake down to 30-35 percent of our total diet calories. But again, we shouldn't attempt to cut fats out completely, and when a diet has less than 30 percent fat it doesn't taste very good and hence will not be followed. Why recommend a diet that will not be eaten?

But There Are Fats—And There Are Fats

The science of nutrition has become very sophisticated. In studying the subject of dietary fats, researchers have distinguished between three different types and have shown a relationship between blood levels of a substance called cholesterol and the level of intake of these individual types of fats. We will go into more detail about the relationship of fats, cholesterol and diet in chapters three and six, but right here three important facts should be mentioned.

First, cholesterol is an organic waxy compound (technically, a higher alcohol) which is found only in foods of animal origin and is made naturally by several body tissues, particularly the liver. In other words, cholesterol is always present in the normally functioning body, despite the nature of one's diet, and it plays an important— an essential—role in the formation of digestive juices, sexual secretions, some connective tissue, and one of the vitamins (vitamin D).

Second, it is now known that different types of fats can influence the levels of blood cholesterol. Specifically, some fats and oils have the ability to raise blood cholesterol levels (the saturated fats), others can lower blood cholesterol levels when they replace some of the saturated fats. These are the unsaturated fats, particularly the polyunsaturated fats. It is important to your health (and to your family's health) that you know the difference between the saturated, polyunsaturated and monounsaturated fats.

Undoubtedly you are already familiar with these words. It's difficult these days to go shopping for margarine, cooking oils and similar products without noticing claims about the type of fat included. *Polyunsaturated* fats tend to lower blood cholesterol when they replace some of the saturated fats. Again, these fats are always of vegetable origin, for instance, soybean, corn, cottonseed, sunflower and safflower oils. They are usually in liquid or soft form. *Saturated* fats, on the other hand, tend to raise blood cholesterol. These latter fats are usually solid in form and of animal origin. For instance, meat fats, whole milk, cream products, butter, and the two vegetable fats—coconut and palm oils. Monounsaturated fats (like olive oil) tend to lower blood cholesterol level when they replace saturated fats, but less so than the polyunsaturated fats.

Third, it has been shown that excessive amounts of cholesterol in the blood, which is, among other things, the result of intake of too many calories with resultant gain in weight and too large an intake of saturated fats in the diet, and too large an intake of foods containing cholesterol, have been linked with atherosclerosis (a type of arteriosclerosis), a disease in which the arteries become narrow and obstructed and pave the way for the real possibility of a heart attack or a cerebral hemorrhage (stroke). It long has been known that cholesterol is one of the ingredients in the mushy deposits, or plaques, that block arteries, but now it has been shown that these blockages can be brought about in every species of laboratory animal by feeding them high-fat, high-cholesterol diets. Monkeys get heart disease similar to that in humans if fed a diet moderately high in saturated fats and cholesterol. Some die very sudden deaths.

This is not to say that eating a great deal of saturated fats and cholesterol is the only underlying cause of heart disease; we know that other things, including hereditary factors, high blood pressure, cigarette smoking, obesity, diabetes, a sedentary life and, no doubt, other factors are involved. But it is clear now that a rich diet, which contributes to the buildup of cholesterol and the associated interference with blood flow and clotting is a critical factor in coronary heart disease.

So what are you going to do about it? We'll get into some of the details on "eating to your heart's content" later, but in talking generally about the fats in our life, it is important to emphasize that we should try to reduce the allover percentage of our diets made up by fats and make an effort to substitute unsaturated, particularly polyunsaturated, fats for about half of the saturated ones. In everyday terms this means emphasizing low-saturated fat and cholesterol main courses such as fish, poultry and veal instead of eating a steady diet of meats such as beef (the main source of saturated fats in our usual diets), using polyunsaturated margarines instead of butter, and eating fewer egg yolks (the yolk of an egg is a highly concentrated form of cholesterol). Egg white contains no cholesterol and is almost pure protein of excellent nutritional quality.

A Look At Vitamins

If you believe everything you read today about vitamins, you'd be convinced that they, alone and preferably in quantity, were magic tablets.

Actually, the name "vitamins," derived from the words "vita" and "amines," suggest that they are life-giving substances, and indeed they are necessary for healthful living and indispensible for the body's many activities. But again, vitamins are only one part of a well-balanced diet. So in making decisions about what type, in what form, and how many vitamins to include in your diet, be advised by your physician, not your next-door neighbor or the "health magazines."

Vitamins have been around since the beginning of time (an E. R. Squibb advertisement once read, "Adam and Eve ate the first vitamins, including the package.") But it is only relatively recent in our history that we learned what vitamins were all about. Actually, if you enjoy a good mystery, the story of vitamins will intrigue you, for the discovery of vitamins has been full of masterful detective work. There's been meticulous tracking down of minute details to find these substances which have so much control of our lives.

Food scientists have solved many vitamin riddles so far. Some have required more high-powered sleuthing than others, and it is likely that there are vitamins yet to be discovered. The last one, vitamin B_{12}, was found some twenty years ago. Solving one vitamin mystery is a monumental accomplishment. It can save hundreds, thousands and more lives. That beats any paperback action!

There is the case of the many Danish children, during World War I, who were bothered by their eyes—they became dry, tearless and their eyelids were swollen and red. Blindness resulted. Through long and thorough observation in experiments with rats, a Danish doctor, Dr. C. E. Bloch, found clues involved with butterfat. The Danes were exporting all their butter to England during the war, leaving only skim milk for their children. Dr. Bloch found that adding whole milk and butter to the children's diets cleared up their eye conditions immediately. After months of research on the magic of butterfat, vitamin A was isolated. It was found to play a part in other eye conditions.

Paralyzed, dying sailors and wobbling, drunklike chickens were symptoms which led to the finding of vitamin B_1 or thiamine. Late in the last century, a medical officer in the Japanese navy tried to find why his sailors were becoming paralyzed and dying. He suspected sanitation at first, but after efforts to remedy this, his sailors remained the same. Finally he noticed that English sailors didn't suffer from the disorder. Long study prompted him to change the Oriental diet of his men from polished rice to whole grains, meat, fish and milk which the English ate. Recovery was immediate.

At the same time a Dutch doctor was trying to seek the cause of the same illness on the island of Java. He thought he had isolated the germ which caused the disease and injected it into chickens to test it. The chickens wobbled when they walked, but then he noticed that even the untested chickens wobbled. Soon the chickens recovered, however. The good doctor traced it to a change in diet of the fowl. They had been switched to a cheaper feed—one of brown, unpolished rice, which made them well. This indicated a dietary change for people too—and the cure attained. Both sets of observations, from the Japanese naval officer and the Dutch doctor, were steps in the discovery of vitamin B_1 or thiamin, the anti-beriberi substance. Just a few of the many examples of nutritional super sleuthing!

It's worth taking a closer look at each of the vitamins that play a role in our lives, keeping in mind that we generally need only a very small amount of each in our daily intake to ensure good health, that these small requirements are easily met by eating a varied, well-balanced diet and that supplementation except in unique situations is unnecessary and may indeed prove harmful to health. In this chapter we'll just introduce you to the cast of vitamins, how they function to keep us healthy and where in your pantry and refrigerator you can find them. Later on in the book we'll deal with the sticky question of vitamin supplements and the fantastic claims which are currently being made about certain "in" vitamins. Later, also, we'll look closely at the dangers of self-prescription of high-dose vitamins. But now, the basics.

First let's consider the group known as the "fat-soluble vitamins," vitamins A, D, E and K, which have in common the fact that they have poor solubility in water and good solubility in fat solvents.

Fat-Soluble Vitamins

Vitamin A

You probably recall from your school nutrition courses that vitamin A is essential for growth, vision and healthy skin. Your mother probably coaxed you into eating your carrots by telling you it would help you see in the dark, and indeed, impaired dark adaptation and night blindness are well-known manifestations of vitamin A deficiency. Without vitamin A, the secretions that formerly bathed the eye dry up, the cornea becomes irritated and eventually vision suffers. (This is what happened to those Danish schoolchildren.) Furthermore, vitamin A is essential for children in promoting their optimal growth. A physician can detect vitamin A deficiency by noting particular problems with the functioning of the central nervous system, a condition which results when soft bones grow faster than spinal bones and in the process, important nerves become pinched.

Where do you find vitamin A? The "direct" form of this vitamin is only found in foods of animal origin. Liver, for instance, is an excellent source. A two-ounce serving of cooked beef liver provides more than 30,000 International Units (IU) of this vitamin. That's six times more vitamin A than you need in a day. Kidney dishes are also an excellent source of vitamin A. Additionally you'll find vitamin A in meat products such as milk, butter and cheese. Remember, while whole milk is a good source of this vitamin, skim milk is not unless it has been fortified (read your labels!).

But your mother was right: carrots and other deep-yellow and dark-green vegetables also will help you meet your vitamin A requirements. In these instances the intake of vitamin A is "indirect." These particular vegetables and fruits supply a yellow pigment called *carotene* from which your body can make vitamin A. Don't be fooled by the dark-green vegetables which look like they don't have the orange-reddish shade which we usually associate with carotenes. In these cases the green pigment chlorophyll masks the presence of the carotene. Even nature has color additives.

You'll have no trouble in getting your necessary amount of vitamin A from eating well-balanced meals, and you needn't worry about getting too much vitamin A from normal dietary sources. But beware of high-dose vitamin A supplements. They could mean trouble.

Vitamin D

Vitamin D is required for the formation of strong bones and teeth and is necessary for the formation of the protein that acts as a carrier for the mineral calcium, facilitating its passage through the intestinal wall. You've heard of the deficiency disease which results from insufficent vitamin D: rickets is characterized by poor calcification of the bones and the victims (inevitably, growing children) have enlarged joints, bowed legs, and knock-knees.

Vitamin D is unique in that you get it not only from the diet, but also your body can produce it from the action of the sun's ultraviolet rays and certain compounds in your skin. Most frequently we get vitamin D from a combination of these sources. It occurs naturally in limited amounts only in animal foods such as eggs, meat, cheese and butter. In our modern diets, however, the richest source of this vitamin is milk which has been fortified with 400 International Units of vitamin D. And of course direct exposure of the skin to sunlight will produce vitamin D for us too.

With regard to supplements of vitamin D, the same warning as was offered for vitamin A must be made: too much of fat-soluble vitamin D from heavy vitamin supplementation builds up in the body and causes problems. You can't get too much vitamin D—or too little—by eating a wide variety of food and/or getting in or out of the sunshine.

Vitamin E

Vitamin E has good public relations managers. Whoever they are, they have managed to convince a great proportion of worldwide eaters that this "super vitamin" can make you sexually young, ease arthritis pains, prevent ulcers and miscarriage, treat cirrhosis of the liver and cancer, improve sperm quality, and generally promote physical endurance. One of the most spectacular claims made by proponents of this vitamin is that it both cures and prevents heart disease. But we're getting ahead of ourselves. Here we're interested in the fact, not the fiction, about vitamin E.

Vitamin E is a fat-soluble chemical in the alcohol family. Its chief function is that of an antioxidant, that is, it inhibits the combination of a substance with oxygen and thus acts as a preservative. Most important, it appears that vitamin E can prevent the oxidation of vitamin A and certain fats, and enables these nutrients to perform their specified roles. In other words, vitamin E protects these nutrients because once they are oxidized they cannot react in their unique ways.

Additionally, it is known that vitamin E plays a protective role with respect to red blood cells. You're right, those activities don't sound anywhere near as exciting as the claim that vitamin E keeps you sexually young! Sorry! But we're sticking here to nutritional facts.

Sources of vitamin E surround us. It is virtually impossible in the modern world for an adult to develop a deficiency of this nutrient. Indeed the early researchers who discovered vitamin E (it was discovered in the mid 1930s and first synthesized in 1938) attempted to learn what happened to laboratory animals who were deprived of it and found that their most difficult task was planning a diet that would cause vitamin E deficiency!

Vitamin K

The fourth fat-soluble vitamin is vitamin K, the so-called "anti-hemorrhagic" vitamin. This vitamin got its letter-designation from the word "koagulation," the Danish spelling. Vitamin K is necessary for blood clotting. But beware! Maybe some day soon someone will try to convince you that the K stands for Kangaroo (well, some people think that vitamin C stands for "colds") and will subsequently recommend that you take large amounts of this vitamin to enlarge and strengthen your hind legs.

Where do you look to find vitamin K? A good source of this vitamin is alfalfa, but this is not yet an important food in our diet. More conventional sources include dark-green, leafy vegetables, liver, egg yolks and soybean oil. It is very unlikely that an individual more than a few days old would develop a deficiency of this vitamin because as soon as the intestinal flora are established, the bacteria in the intestine produce their own vitamin K, a good bit of which we absorb. In fact this is our main source of this vitamin. In other words, we don't have to depend on outside sources for our vitamin K.

Water Soluble Vitamins

Vitamin C (Ascorbic Acid)

The history of vitamin C is closely linked with that of its deficiency disease, scurvy. Scurvy was the scourge of sailors who took voyages of many weeks without fresh fruit. It wasn't until 1747 that a Scottish physician, Dr. James Lind showed that scurvy could be cured or prevented by consumption of citrus fruits. This discovery, far before the identification of the vitamin itself, led to the inclusion of limes in the sailors' diets. The nickname "limeys" in referring to British soldiers is related directly to the use of that citrus fruit in their travels.

The exact functions of vitamin C in the human diet are not fully understood. One recognized function of this vitamin is in the formation of connective tissue that serves to cement the cells and tissues together, and thus, among other things, allows wounds to heal. Do you recall our experimenting physician, William Starr, in 1770, who complained of "small ulcers on the inside of my cheeks, particularly near a bad tooth; the gums of the upper jaw of the same side were swelled and red and bled when pressed with the finger"? Here, although he didn't know it at the time, Dr. Starr was describing the classical signs of vitamin C deficiency.

Citrus fruits and juices have become almost synonymous with vitamin C, and it is well-known that these are excellent sources of this vitamin. Vitamin C deficiency in this country today is very rare, so eat your citrus and don't worry about it.

And what about colds and vitamin C? It hasn't much to do with either the prevention or treatment of the common cold, despite what our two-time Nobel Prize winner Professor Linus Pauling says. A recent unbiased review in the *Journal of the American Medical Association* concluded: "The unrestricted use of ascorbic acid (vitamin C) for these purposes (prevention and treatment of the common cold) cannot be advocated on the basis of the evidence currently available." We look more closely at the alleged vitamin C-cold link in the next chapter.

Vitamin B Complex

The various B vitamins play a number of important roles. Among other things, they are involved in maintaining healthy skin (especially around the mouth, nose and eyes) and well-functioning nervous system, working with carbohydrates for energy in the body. The summary table will give you the details about where to find which particular B vitamin you are looking for at the moment, but generally, if your diet includes milk, whole-grain cereals and breads, meats (occasionally liver), and vegetables, you have no need to be concerned about getting enough of any B vitamin.

Take note of vitamin B_{12} (for those who like big words, the technical name cyanocobalamin should be part of your vocabulary—if you can pronounce it). Yes, this is another nasty chemical, but so are all nutrients. It can only be found in animal products, particularly meats. If vegetarians exclude products such as eggs and milk from their diet, in addition to direct meat sources, they will have a problem. But we'll go into techniques of balancing the vegetarian diet in chapter five.

Minerals

What are minerals? They are the substances you have remaining in food after the protein, carbohydrates, fat, vitamins, and water are removed. And we need minerals daily, if only in very small amounts. The minerals you should know something about include iron, calcium, iodide and fluoride, and for some people, sodium and potassium.

Iron is an essential component of hemoglobin, the pigment in the red blood cells which carry oxygen from the lungs to the tissues. Because the body has an amazing capacity to preserve iron, the nutritional needs of healthy males and also of women beyond reproductive age is very small. Reproductive-age women, however, must make up the iron they lose during menstruation and childbirth. And children have relatively high needs because of their rapid growth which not only increases their body size, but also their blood volume.

Iron is present in a variety of foods of both plant and animal origin. In many foods there is a considerable variation in the value of iron content according to the soil conditions in which the food is raised. Rich food sources for iron include meat (especially liver), egg yolk, beans and peas. However, many other common foods such as green leafy vegetables, whole-grain and enriched cereals, vegetables, certain fruits and fish are good sources of iron. Milk, both human and cow's milk, contrary to the notion that it is the "perfect food," is a poor source of iron.

Both *calcium* and *phosphorus* are known for their contribution to the growth and maintenance of bones and teeth. Additionally, calcium is necessary for blood clotting, healing of wounds and broken bones, and the normal functioning of the heart. The nervous system does not work properly when calcium levels in the blood are abnormal.

A great variety of foods, such as whole-grain cereal products, leafy vegetables, legumes and nuts contain calcium, with particularly rich sources being milk and cheese. Sardines and other small fish in which the bones are eaten are other important sources of calcium. Phosphorus is needed in combination with calcium for healthy bones and teeth, and the needs for this mineral are met by eating calcium-rich foods such as milk and cheese. Meats, chicken, and fish are also good sources of phosphorus.

The most important fact you should know about the mineral *iodine* is that a deficiency of it can cause *goiter,* that is, a swelling of the thyroid gland. Seafoods on the whole are rich in iodide, and dairy products, eggs and some vegetables may be good sources. But the most practical way to avoid a deficiency of iodide is to use iodized salt. Again, read the labels! You'll notice that salt that does not have iodide is labeled "This salt does not supply iodide, a necessary nutrient." This label is now required by federal law.

Fluoride is an essential mineral nutrient because it is required for maximum resistance to dental cavities, particularly in the young, and for resistance to osteoporosis, a chronic disease of aging which is responsible for much pain, commonly in the back, and for the ease with which bones frequently break in the elderly. But fluoride is not readily found in food, and it is thus essential that trace amounts of it be included in our water supply. Most minerals evoke virtually no emotional response when they are being discussed, but this certainly is not true for fluoride. We'll get into more of the specifics of how fluoridated water is an essential component of good dental health in the next chapter, but what is critical here is the recognition of the importance of fluoride in the diet for both young and old, and the practical observation that we're not going to get as much as we need for good health unless the well-established public health principle of water fluoridation is widely implemented.

There are other minerals necessary in our diet: chloride, cobalt, copper, magnesium, manganese, molybdenum, potassium, chromium, selenium, sodium, sulphur, zinc, lead, mercury, tin and other metals (some of which are mentioned in the chart), but here it is sufficient to emphasize that, as a total group, minerals are available in fruits, vegetables, milk, eggs, cereal and water, and almost all foods, with the exception of granulated sugar and various oils and fats, contribute to a well-varied intake of all our essential minerals.

Water

If we had been listing components of the human diet by order of priority, water would not be described after proteins, carbohydrates, fats, vitamins and minerals. It would be the very first on the list for survival. People can survive for much longer periods of time when any other nutrient is eliminated from the diet. We can't survive without water. Water stands next to air as the most important substance for the maintenance of life.

What does water do except play the role as a refreshing libation? Water is necessary for all chemical reactions that occur in our bodies. It is needed for the transport of nutrients, for blood, for regulation of body temperature and for elimination of body wastes.

"Drink six to eight glasses of water a day" goes the adage. And it's a physiologically accurate rule of thumb to follow and adapt as necessary. More specifically, we need about one liter (a little more than a quart) for each 1000 Calories we eat. That would mean between two and two and one-half liters of water. But again, the requirements for water intake vary by the nature of the environment you're living in and your physical activity. You hardly need to be reminded that you need more water during the hot summer months to replace that being released by your temperature control mechanism. And after strenuous activity on the tennis courts, a cool, tall drink looks very appealing.

You meet your requirements for water in other ways than by

filling a glass at your kitchen tap or taking advantage of your local water fountain. Water is present in subtle forms. Bread, for instance, seems dry, but it is actually 35 percent water. Most fruits have a water content of over 90 percent. Lettuce is more than 95 percent water. The next time you take a bite out of a banana, a fruit which hardly seems juicy at all, remember that it is about 75 percent water.

Solid food in the average diet contributes 25-50 percent of body water needs each day. Liquids supply a little less than half of the total needed, and the remainder of water utilized by the body is provided daily on an internal basis as a result of water released during metabolism—the utilization of food.

Calories!

Here you are well into a book on nutrition, and we haven't even defined the most popular (or unpopular, depending on your point of view) nutritional topic of all. Calories!

Calories compete with the weather as a popular topic of conversation; nearly all of us talk about them. And many of us are deceived by them because we don't really know what calories have to do with getting fat, or with "fattening foods," or with body fat. What is a calorie, where does it come from, and how is it used?

Despite the fact that this is in the "know thy nutrient" section, a calorie is not a nutrient or a food. It is a unit for measuring energy, like pounds and quarts are measuring units. The calorie is the unit which expresses how much energy value there is in a food, or how much energy is expended in a particular body process.

The body needs energy for everything it does, like digesting food, breathing, or walking. How does it obtain this energy? By taking the carbohydrate, fat, or protein of any food we eat and combining it with oxygen (in the body cells). This reaction produces a certain number of calories of energy. Calories of energy are the fuel for body processes, as gasoline is the fuel that provides energy for a car.

In other words, the calorie value of one's foods supports the calorie cost of daily living. When we say that "a slice of bread is sixty Calories," we mean that it has an energy value of sixty Calories, and that, therefore, it can provide sixty Calories for a particular activity, like a brisk fifteen-minute walk.

Notice that we occasionally spell calories with a capital "C."

The reason is that the Calories in a specific food or required for exercise are kilocalories—that is, 1,000 little calories. Thus we use Calories (kilocalories) when mentioning the Calories of a food or exercise and calories when simply referring to calories in general.

Since foods vary in composition, they vary in the number of calories they yield. However, they do not vary in kinds of calories. *One hundred Calories from one food has exactly the same fuel value as 100 Calories from any other food,* whether that food is grapefruit, jam or ham, carbohydrate, protein, fat, or even alcohol. And don't let anyone convince you otherwise!

Usually for an adult all the food calories that are eaten (or drunk) in a day should equal all the energy calories used up in that day's activities. If your car burns one gallon of gas every fifteen miles, you must plan on six gallons for a ninety-mile excursion. More than this is unnecessary, and less causes trouble. The daily need for calories needs the same kind of careful calculation.

A certain basic number of calories are required to support basic body processes (referred to as Basal Metabolism), such as the beating of the heart, breathing, and maintaining a normal body temperature. In addition, extra calories are demanded for each activity and for special conditions such as growth or pregnancy, and all of these are influenced by other factors, such as size, age, sex, physical condition, and climate. The sum total of all these items determines how many calories an individual should eat or drink each day.

If a persons eats less than this, weight is lost because the body consumes its own fat as a source of energy. If a person eats too much, weight is gained because there is no effective way to eliminate the extra calories. *All* foods are turned into calories of energy for body use, and therefore all of these calories must count in the day's total. If there is more than enough, the surplus is turned into fat and deposited somewhere in the body, and how nice it would be if we could control the places in the body where this extra fat is deposited. But alas, we cannot.

So it is the extra calories of food, over and above the daily requirement, which put on excess pounds of fat. Some foods contain few calories, some many, but they only become "fattening" if the day's total food and drink intake is more than the body engine uses. The secret of caloric success is to make sure that intake and output are in balance!

So far we've been looking at the individual categories of nutrients that make up good nutrition. But before we turn to the practical application of these nutritional guidelines in everyday meal planning (chapter three), let's pause for a moment to see how all these substances work together to keep us happy and healthy.

TO EAT IS HUMAN, TO DIGEST DIVINE

In the kitchen, or at the table, if we put too much sugar into tea or coffee, we may not like it, but the sugar is there to stay. Or, once flour has been beaten into a batter, not all the cook's men can get it out again.

Yet put one morsel into your mouth, and it is a very different story. Each bite begins a whole series of amazing reactions, whose purpose is to split all foods into their individual nutrients. For instance, the sugar that was added to coffee, or that is hidden in fruit, or the flour that was put into cake must be freed from the rest of the food before they can be used as sources of body energy.

All foods undergo this change and completely lose their identity. Milk or meat, fruit or honey or cane sugar simply cannot travel from cell to cell, depositing their valuables. They must be split and altered by digestion before their individual nutrients can carry out their life-giving functions.

Digestion divides every liquid, every solid, every mixture, into its content of the six basic nutrients we just discussed: protein, carbohydrate, fat, vitamins, minerals, and water. And this is only one step. Afterwards the nutrients are further subdivided into their basic components, such as amino acids, fatty acids, and the simple sugar known as glucose. After all of this is completed, then at last foods are ready to supply nutrition for the millions of body cells.

Digestion is one of the many complicated body activities which we take for granted. How often do we wonder about the fate of the grilled cheese sandwich we had for lunch? Well, in case you ever do, be aware that the processes that determine what happens to the bread, cheese and whatever else you had in there had begun even before you put it in your mouth. Just thinking about eating it or smelling the food starts up the transmission of a key message. Some people can't even read a book about food without triggering a mouth watering response! Is your mouth watering now? Notice what happens next time you are really hungry and look at a picture of a juicy, sizzling cheeseburger.

Once you put the food in your mouth, it meets up with the enzymes in saliva. These particular enzymes specialize in starting the digestion of starch. And when you swallow the food, it quickly arrives in the highly acid environment of the stomach where it is churned around for some time (a half-hour to two or three hours, depending on the composition of the food—the more fat the longer in the stomach). Finally, your grilled cheese sandwich, or anything else for that matter, is reduced to a semifluid state known as chyme.

Then on to the small intestine where the acidified food is neutralized and mixed with bile. This is the fluid manufactured from the liver and stored in the gallbladder, and helps to cut or emulsify the fat into globules to facilitate its absorption. Also, fats, carbohydrates and proteins are acted on by many, many specialized enzymes which are provided by your very own enzyme factory, the pancreas. And the small intestine itself gets into the act by providing its own enzymes. As the food residues reach the far end of the small intestine and the beginning of the large intestine, even our own "friendly bacteria" break down various nutrients. Passage of the food from the time we swallow and on down the gastrointestinal tract is by a series of contractions of muscles in the wall of the intestine, a process known as peristalsis.

Don't let anyone talk you into eating raw or uncooked foods for the reason that they will provide you with needed enzymes. Any enzymes present in raw foods are quickly destroyed by the strong acid of the stomach, and our major enzyme factory—the pancreas— makes many, many times more enzymes than might have been present in raw foods.

Well, we told you it was complicated! And we're not through with discussing the transformation of our grilled cheese sandwich. Once the lunch has been broken up into simple sugars, amino acids and fatty acids, the basic particles, alone or in combination, are ready to be absorbed into the bloodstream through the fingerlike projections of the small intestines—the villi. And everything that can be absorbed is absorbed. The residue of undigested material, commonly called "roughage" or fiber (to be discussed next), promotes muscle tone and stimulates the peristalsis in the intestine to speed digestion. Eventually all waste materials enter the large intestine where they are stored until they are eliminated some eighteen or more hours after the food first entered the digestive tract.

Roughage* or Fiber

Roughage in the diet, once a topic pursued by everyone with real gusto, gave way to talk about the more sophisticated-sounding elements of the diet such as vitamins and, more recently, polyunsaturated fats. But roughage is currently having a renaissance via renewed interest in the fiber content of the diet.

Roughage has not lost its importance or its useful function in your diet. Roughage is the indigestible material found in food: in vegetables, it is called cellulose and forms the skeleton of most plants; in cereals it is the bran portion; in fruits the skin; in animals, it is the connective tissue—the tough parts of meat that are almost impossible to chew.

Even though it contributes little if anything to the purely nutritive value of the diet, roughage or fiber does aid the mechanics of digestion. Its presence in the intestinal tract provides a medium for growth of bacteria that help the body synthesize certain nutrients— vitamin K, for example. Most people, especially bran eaters, know that roughage—or bulk, as it is sometimes called—helps rid the body of waste materials. Actually, bulk or fiber is a better name than roughage, for it is not "rough" on one's intestines.

Whole-grain cereals, nuts, fruits, and vegetables provide most of the roughage or fiber in the ordinary diet. Bran, the outer layer of cereal grains, is a rich source of fiber. Relatively large amounts are also found in fruits, such as berries, and in fruits where the skins are consumed, such as plums and grapes, also in most vegetables. Milk, eggs, cheese, and highly refined foods such as white flour and sugar have no roughage or fiber.

Of considerable interest to most of us is the eye and taste appeal that roughage-containing foods lend to our meals: tossed green salads, fresh berries, carrots, sliced tomatoes, broccoli—to mention a few. The cook in a family with an ulcer-stricken member quickly learns how many foods contain roughage. He or she knows and appreciates how challenging it is to plan appetizing meals when roughage is limited, but even here modern medicine is backing away from the idea that a low-fiber diet is desirable for those with ulcers.

Generally, however, the person who consumes a well-balanced diet

---

*We'll have more to say about "high fiber" diets in our section dealing with nutrition and cancer.

selected from a wide variety of foods will get enough roughage, particularly if some whole-grain breads, cereals and fruits with edible skins are eaten. A few people, for medical reasons, need more or less than average. Frequently, the common type of constipation can be treated and prevented by a diet moderately high in bulk-producing residues. Such a diet may need to include stewed fruits (prunes or apricots) two or three times a day and a bran cereal once a day.

* * * * *

So there you have them: the basic facts of nutrition. Take time to *digest them*, then move on to see how you can put the basics to work for you.

SPECIFIC NUTRIENTS AND THEIR FUNCTIONS

Where You Can Find Them	What They Do
Protein	Is constituent of all body cells.
Meat, fish, poultry, egg white, milk, cheese.	Needed for: structure of red blood cells (hemoglobin); antibodies to fight infection and disease; and enzymes and hormones to regulate body processes.
Dried beans and peas, peanut butter, nuts, bread and cereal have nutritionally incomplete proteins but are adequate if served with milk or eggs, or meat.	Needed for growth, maintenance and repair of tissue. Regulates amount of water present in the spaces between body cells.
Carbohydrates	Primary source of energy for the body.
Flours, cereals, breads, cakes, crackers, rice, noodles, macaroni, spaghetti, sugars, syrups, jellies, honey and jams.	Primary energy source for the brain and nervous tissue.
Some fruits and vegetables such as dried fruits, sweetened fruits, dried legumes, potatoes, corn, lima beans and bananas.	Protects protein—spares the body from using protein to meet energy needs.
Cellulose and fibers.	Complex carbohydrate is needed for bulk and proper elimination, and the normal growth of bacteria in the lower intestine.

3 *Fats*

Fat from beef, lamb, and pork; butter, margarine, lard, salad oil, hydrogenated shortening; cream, milk, cheese (except those made with skim milk); fried foods, pastries, chocolates, and rich desserts.

Provide concentrated form of energy for the body.

Carry the fat-soluble vitamins A, D and E into the body; provide protection for various vital organs and insulation for the body; increase palatability of food; provide "satisfaction"—delay onset of hunger.

4 *Vitamin A*

Liver, kidney (excellent sources), egg yolk, dark-green leafy and deep-yellow vegetables, tomatoes, butter, fortified margarine, whole milk and cheese made from whole milk and fortified skim milk.

Needed for growth, healthy skin, bones, and teeth, particularly for children.

Helps maintain good vision, especially in poor light.

Helps body resist infection.

5 *Vitamin D*

Fortified milk, egg yolk, liver, fish (herring, sardines, tuna, salmon).

With direct sunlight on the skin the body can manufacture its own.

Needed for the absorption and utilization of calcium and phosphorus.

Needed for healthy bones and sound teeth.

6 *Vitamin E*

Green leafy vegetables, nuts, legumes, salad oils, shortenings, margarines, meat, fish, milk, eggs and many other sources.

Helps protect vitamin A and polyunsaturated fatty acids.

Protects red blood cells. (Has nothing to do with sex or heart disease!)

7 *Vitamin K*

Synthesized naturally by bacteria in the human intestinal tract. Smallish amounts in green leaves of spinach, kale and cabbage; cauliflower, pork liver.

Promotes normal blood clotting.

8 *Vitamin C (Ascorbic Acid)*

Citrus fruits, strawberries, tomatoes, cantaloupe, broccoli, raw green vegetables, cabbage, boiled potato, canned or frozen citrus fruit juices.

Needed for building the material that holds cells together. Needed for health of teeth, gums and blood vessels. Helps resist infection and aids in healing wounds (but is not effective in the prevention or treatment of the common cold). Helps synthesize hormones to regulate body functions, improves iron absorption.

Ϥ *Vitamin B Group:*

Riboflavin (B₂)

Milk and cheese are the best sources.

Liver, kidney and heart, other meats, eggs, green leafy vegetables, enriched breads and cereals.

A constituent of many enzymes needed to use protein, fats and carbohydrates for energy and building tissues.

Maintains healthy skin, especially around the mouth, nose and eyes.

Thiamine (B₁)

Whole-grain products or enriched breads and cereals.

Meats (especially pork), poultry, fish.

Liver, dry beans and peas, soybeans, peanuts, egg yolk.

Helps to use carbohydrates for energy in the body.

Helps maintain healthy nervous system.

Niacin

Poultry, meats, fish and organ meats are the best sources.

Peanuts, peanut butter, legumes, dark-green leafy vegetables, potatoes, whole-grain or enriched breads, cereals.

Needed for healthy nervous system, healthy skin, normal digestion.

Helps cells use oxygen to release energy.

Needed to use protein in the body.

Needed for normal growth.

Pyridoxine (B₆)

Meats (especially pork and the glandular meats), lamb, veal, liver, kidney, wheat germ, whole-grain cereals, soybeans, peanuts, corn.

Prevents certain forms of anemia.

Needed for normal utilization of copper and iron.

Pantothenic Acid

Meats, liver, kidney, heart, fish, eggs, vegetables, legumes, whole grains.

Breakdown of carbohydrates, fats, and proteins for the production of energy.

Synthesis of amino acids, fatty acids, sterols, and steroid hormones.

Vitamin B₁₂ (Cyanocobalamin)

Provided only by foods of animal origin: meats (especially liver and kidney), fish, milk, eggs, cheese. Does not occur in fruits, vegetables, or cereals—so, vegetarians beware!

Needed for production of red blood cells in bone marrow.

Needed for building new proteins in the body.

Needed for normal functioning of nervous tissue.

Folacin or Folic Acid

Variety of foods of animal and vegetable origin, particularly glandular meats, such as liver, but also in green leafy vegetables, many fruits, eggs, and whole-grain cereals.

Necessary for the development of red blood cells.

Needed for normal metabolism of carbohydrates, proteins, and fats.

Biotin

Meats, egg yolk, legumes, nuts.

Interrelated with functions of others in the vitamin B group.

Minerals

10 *Iron*

Liver, lean meats, poultry, shellfish, egg yolk, clams, oysters.

Green leafy vegetables, whole-grain and enriched cereals and breads, legumes and nuts, molasses. Certain fruits such as peaches, apricots, prunes, grapes, raisins.

Needed for normal metabolism of carbohydrates, proteins, and fats.

Needed to form hemoglobin which carries oxygen from the lungs to the body cells.

A component of many, many enzymes.

11 *Calcium*

Milk, cheese. (Hard water.)

Greens: turnip, collards, Kale, mustard.

Ice cream, cottage cheese (less calcium than regular cheese), broccoli, oysters, shrimp, salmon, clams, cabbage.

Needed for structure of bones and teeth.

Needed for healthy nerves and muscle activity.

Essential in blood clotting.

Needed in healing wounds and broken bones.

Phosphorus

Meats, milk, cheese, ice cream, meat, poultry, fish, whole-grain cereals, nuts, legumes.

Dietary deficiency unlikely if diet contains enough protein and calcium.

Needed in combination with calcium for bones and teeth.

Needed for enzymes used in energy metabolism.

Regulates the balance between acids and bases in the body.

12 *Iodide*

Iodized salt is best source.

Seafoods and foods grown along the seacoast.

Needed to make the hormone thyroxine, which regulates the use of energy in the body.

Prevents goiter.

Fluoride

Fluoridated water.

Promotion of good dental health, prevention of osteoporosis.

Copper

Meats, particularly liver, shellfish, nuts, raisins, dried legumes, cereal, cocoa, chocolate.

Synthesis of hemoglobin and metabolism of iron.

Maintenance of normal blood vessels.

Magnesium

Whole-grain cereals, potatoes, nuts, legumes, meat. (Hard water).

Dietary deficiency unlikely.

Needed for structure of bones and teeth.

Helps transmit nerve impulses.

Helps muscle contraction.

Activates enzymes needed for carbohydrate and energy metabolism.

Potassium

Citrus fruits, cantaloupe, bananas, apricots, other fresh fruits, fruit juices, vegetables, meat, fish and cereals.

Ample amounts in well-balanced diet.

Aids the synthesis of protein. Helps maintain fluid balance.

Required for healthy nerves and muscles.

Needed for enzyme reactions.

Sodium (Salt)

Table salt, meat, fish, poultry, milk, eggs.

In foods where salt is a preservative (ham, bacon, olives, fish).

Helps maintain fluid balance.

Keeps balance of acids and bases in body.

Helps in the absorption of other nutrients including glucose.

Zinc

Green leafy foods, fruit, whole grains, meats and vegetables.

Helps in wound healing. Component of many enzymes.

Essential for normal growth and development.

Water

Water acts in many ways to keep us healthy. First, it is a practical medium for transporting nutrients to the various cells of the body and for removing the cellular waste products. Second, water serves as a cushioning device since it is not readily compressible and acts additionally as a lubricant in body movement. Third, water is an essential compound in the chemical reactions of digestion, breaking down carbohydrates, splitting glycerol from fatty acids, among other processes. Fourth, water gives structure to the body, retaining the shape of cells. Some 40 percent of body weight is water located within cells. Fifth, water serves as a temperature-regulating substance: the evaporation of water from the lungs and skin removes heat from the body. If you want to demonstrate your water loss from your lungs, breathe into a glass. There you will have your evidence.

Chapter Three

Biting, Chewing, Swallowing and Digesting Your Way to Good Health

WE'VE GOT YOUR NUMBER!
SPOTLIGHT ON THE BASIC FOUR

Is there a magic formula for healthful eating? Yes, there is, and it goes something like this: eat a variety of foods and don't eat too much of anything.

Why should a diet be balanced? Because the right amounts of the right foods make a big difference in one's life and one's well-being. Because a balanced diet builds health and vigor.

All through life, cells, tissues, and organs depend on food for materials to repair and rebuild themselves. If the food is inadequate, the body is bound to suffer.

This means that you yourself can do a great deal to make good health, or better health, a reality for yourself and the members of your family. You can do this simply by choosing a balanced diet.

Yet many people, even in the United States, do not eat what they should. Some are overstuffed with food. Still others are overstuffed with pills. Thousands more skimp on the nutrients that build health.

This is not because food is scarce or knowledge lacking. Nutritionists have found that some fifty nutrients are indispensable for everything we do: breathing, eating, moving, thinking, even resting. Experts know which foods contain these nutrients. Farmers and merchants supply these foods in greater abundance than the world has ever known.

But you do the eating. You won't have all the necessary nutrients unless you plan meals that are not only appetizing but are also healthful.

This need not be difficult or complicated. You don't need expensive items, or special foods, or supplements from the "health-food" stores. You don't have to jiggle weights or memorize figures.

All you require is a balanced diet. This is your guide to the right amounts of all the food groups, plus water, roughage and calories. The balanced diet is the simple, safe and sure way to eat well, to control weight, and to feel well.

In the 1940s the United States Department of Agriculture devised what they called the "Basic Seven" to explain the variety of foods needed in the diet for good nutrition. They listed milk, meats, citrus fruits, green and yellow vegetables, other fruits and vegetables, bread and cereals, and butter or margarine. Actually this list was a condensed version of the "Basic Eleven" which ruled the nutritional world earlier in the century.

In an effort to simplify the nutritional guidelines even further, we at Harvard's Department of Nutrition designed and published in the *Journal of the American Dietetic Association* in 1958 what we called the "Basic Four" as a guide to variety and balance. These four basic food groups can bring strength, energy and good nutrition to every individual who wants to be healthy. And who doesn't? A few months after we published our Basic Four, the USDA designed their own Basic Four. Fortunately they are both essentially the same—and they offer us a convenient way to plan our meals throughout the day.

Group 1: Dairy Products.

First is milk or things made from milk. Nearly everyone should have some milk or milk product every day for protein of high nutritional value, calcium and phosphorus and certain vitamins. The recommended amount of milk per day varies by age. Generally you should be guided by the following:

Children under 8 or 9 years of age	1-2 glasses
Teen-agers	3-4 glasses
Adults	1 or more glasses
Pregnant women	3 or more glasses
Nursing mothers	4 or more glasses

You can tell from the above that milk is particularly important during the childhood and teen-age years and during pregnancy and lactation, but remember that you wouldn't want to go much above the recommended amounts at any age lest your dairy foods crowd out other good foods. This would defeat the "magic formula" of variety in food consumption.

In general you can substitute other milk products for milk, evaluating other products from the point of view of how large a serving it would take to replace a given amount of milk. For instance, a one-inch cube of cheddar-type cheese or one-half cup of yogurt is equal to one-half a cup of milk; one-half a cup of cottage cheese, or ice cream, or ice milk is approximately equal to one-third cup of milk. Take these milk "substitute" values into consideration when planning your daily intake of food from the dairy products group.

But let's pause for a moment to take a look at that all-important food, milk, and some of the (incorrect) rumors that are currently being spread about it.

"Milk is good for children but bad for adults," "It's poisonous as nicotine for grown-ups," some self-proclaimed nutritionists are saying. "It has large amounts of cholesterol, the substance suspected of helping to cause the buildup of fatty deposits in arteries," say others. Except for the last half of the last statement, all of the above is pure rubbish.

Milk and its products are good for most children, most adults, and most oldsters. Why? The protein of milk is of excellent nutritional quality (none better) and is generous in quantity. One eight-ounce glass of milk provides about eight grams of protein. This is more protein than there is in one egg and about half as much as there is in a three-ounce serving of meat. Milk is the only good source of calcium in our diets, the best source of the B vitamin riboflavin, a good source of many other B vitamins, of vitamin A, and most milk today is fortified with vitamin D.

What are milk's nutritional shortcomings? Iron, the B vitamin niacin, and fluoride, but there are few foods which approach milk in its overall nutritional value.

What about its cholesterol content? A glass of whole milk provides about 25 milligrams of cholesterol. The same amount of low-fat milk would have half that amount and skim milk essentially none. Compare those figures with 250 milligrams of cholesterol in a single average egg yolk!

Why do we suggest milk for adults in reasonable quantity? Because of the prevalence of osteoporosis (porous, weak bones) among adults, particularly in women after the menopause. And what is a reasonable quantity? One to two glasses a day or its equivalent in ice cream or cheese.

But to get the most out of the mineral calcium in milk as far as "bone health" is concerned, it is necessary to have a good source of the mineral nutrient fluoride. So while you are drinking your milk, make sure your community is fluoridating your water!

Group 2: Meats

In addition to meat (beef, veal, pork, variety meats such as liver, heart and kidney), foods in this group include fish, poultry, eggs, cheese, dried beans and peas, nuts (including peanuts and peanut butter) and lentils.

Two servings daily are desirable to ensure that you get adequate amounts of protein, iron and some of the vitamins. One of those servings should be meat or fish or poultry. One may be an egg or an ounce of cheese. Vegetarians who prefer not to consume meats but will eat animal products can readily get protein of good nutritional quality and sufficient quantity by consuming extra milk, cheese, and eggs.

Group 3: Bread and Cereal Products

Enriched or whole-grain bread and cereals provide energy-giving carbohydrates, many minerals and vitamins and are actually also a good source of protein. Variety in cereal proteins, particularly if consumed in the same meal with a small amount of animal protein, such as milk on breakfast cereals, assures one of protein of excellent nutritional quality.

Specifically, "Group 3" includes breads, cooked cereals, ready-to-eat cereals, cornmeal, crackers, flours, grits, macaroni and spaghetti, noodles, rice, rolled oats, and other baked goods if made with whole-grain or enriched flour. With a list like that you have quite a selection to choose from! The whole-grain and bran-containing cereals are good sources of fiber.

Generally we recommend that you choose four servings or more daily. You count as a serving one slice of bread, one ounce of ready-to-eat cereal, one-half to three-quarters cup of cooked cereal, corn-meal, grits, macaroni, noodles, rice or spaghetti. Bread and cereal products are good for you! Don't be afraid to include them in your diet, if only in moderation. They are no more fattening than other foods and less so than foods with generous amounts of fat such as meats.

Group 4: Vegetables and Fruit

Four servings daily will supply you with vitamins, minerals, and fiber (roughage). One serving should contain vitamin C. Good sources include any citrus fruits or juices, orange, grapefruit, or tangerine, tomato, cantaloupe, guava, mango, papaya, fresh straw-berries, broccoli, Brussels sprouts, and green peppers. Fair sources of vitamin C include other fruits, watermelon, asparagus tips, raw cabbage, collards, garden cress, kale, mustard greens, boiled potatoes and sweet potatoes (preferably cooked in their jackets), spinach or turnip greens.

And at least four times a week you should include a dark-green or yellow vegetable for carotene from which we can make vitamin A. In addition to dark-green and deep-yellow vegetables, you can find carotene in apricots, broccoli, cantaloupe, carrots, kale, pumpkins, spinach, sweet potatoes, turnip greens and winter squash among other vegetables. Count as "one serving" one-half cup of vegetables or fruit of the portion normally served, like one medium potato or half a medium grapefruit.

The avocado is a unique fruit often misunderstood in that some think it is "full of" cholesterol and fat. Like other fruits and vege-tables it has *no* cholesterol; the latter is only in animal foods. The avocado does have more fat than most other fruits and vegetables, an average of 16 percent, but most of the fat (more than 80 percent) is unsaturated, the kind we are trying to increase in our diets. Avo-cados are also excellent sources of vitamins A, E, many of the other vitamins, minerals, and it contains 2 to 3 percent protein, a value far higher than other fruits. The avocado is eaten uncooked with no opportunity for destruction of nutrients from overcooking. In fact, the avocado is a "natural convenience food," tasty, and highly nutritious.

The Basic Four Food Groups are the original health foods! In mentioning them we have stated several servings of "this and that," but, and an important but, adjust the size of the servings to reach the weight you desire, and remember you "beef up" the calories if you smother your vegetables with hollandaise or other fatty sauces and your fruits with cream!

Other Foods

Have we covered everything in the Basic Four? From the nutritional point of view, if you eat a *variety* of foods within each category, you will be eating your way to good health.

But to round out our meals, meet energy needs, and get the palatability we all desire, almost everyone will use some foods not specified in the four food groups: sugars, margarine and other fats, and be sure to include some polyunsaturated fats. Is it okay to eat foods that don't appear on the Basic Four list? Is it okay to enjoy a dry martini, snacks, sauces and stuffings? The answer is an emphatic "yes" but with the all-important qualifier that "fun foods" (actually this is an imprecise term because we mentioned liquor which is not technically a food, although it does provide a generous amount of calories) should never under any circumstances prevent us from getting our share from these four vital food categories.

READ THE LABEL BEFORE YOU PUT IT ON THE TABLE

An understanding of the Basic Four should help you plan and eat healthy nutritious meals, meals that are not only delicious but keep you looking, feeling and functioning at your peak. But there is another tool you have in wise nutrition planning: the new nutritional labels that you now see on many foods.

U. S. RDA is one set of initials which should become familiar to every consumer interested in nutrition and good health. That includes you! The initials stand for "United States Recommended Daily Allowances." These are the amounts of vitamins, minerals and other nutrients from food recommended for a person to eat every day to stay healthy.

Actually there are three RDA'S floating around today. The best known, and the one that will be used on most nutritional-information panels and on most vitamin-mineral supplements, is for adults and children over age four. The second one is for infants and children under four. The third is for pregnant women or women who are nursing their babies.

Table 1

U.S. Recommended Daily Allowances
(U.S. RDA)

Protein	
Protein quality equal to or greater than casein	**45 grams**
Protein quality less than casein	**65 grams**
Vitamin A	**5,000 International Units**
Vitamin C (ascorbic acid)	**60 milligrams**
Thiamine (vitamin B_1)	**1.5 milligrams**
Riboflavin (vitamin B_2)	**1.7 milligrams**
Niacin	**20 Milligrams**
Calcium	**1.0 gram**
Iron	**18 milligrams**
Vitamin D	400 international Units
Vitamin E	30 International Units
Vitamin B_6	2.0 milligrams
Folic acid (folacin)	0.4 milligram
Vitamin B_{12}	6 micrograms
Phosphorus	1.0 gram
Iodine	150 micrograms
Magnesium	400 milligrams
Zinc	15 milligrams
Copper	2 milligrams
Biotin	0.3 milligram
Pantothenic acid	10 milligrams

The nutrients in bold type *must* appear on nutrition labels. The other nutrients *may* appear.

RDA's are amounts of vitamins and minerals plus protein estimated to be needed by both sexes throughout the life cycle. These
allowances will maintain good nutrition in essentially all healthy
persons in the United States and other developed countries under
current living conditions. They are designed to allow a generous
margin of safety above the average requirement. In other words, as
they are not minimum requirements, you won't be in nutritional
trouble if you don't meet the RDA for each nutrient every day, but
it's a good idea to head in that direction.

You'll notice in Table 1 that RDA's are measured either in IU's
(International Units), which are the standards nutritionists work
with, or else in grams, milligrams or micrograms. What you will
see on your labels, however, will be the percentages of each RDA
you will be treating yourself to by eating a defined serving of that
particular product.

What about the other thirty-some nutrients not included in the
list of twenty nutrients? One is likely to obtain these others from a
selection of foods that supply the RDA's and calories in adequate
amounts.

Today's food labels are required on all foods that are enriched and
fortified and foods for which a nutritional claim is made. Other food
labels may voluntarily contain nutrition information. But let's get
specific. Let's say you are serving some raisin bran which makes the
claim "fortified with eight essential vitamins." Its nutritional information label might look something like this:

NUTRITIONAL INFORMATION PER SERVING

Serving size: 1 oz. (about ½ cup)
Servings per package: 15

	Cereal Alone	With ½ cup Vitamin D Fortified Whole Milk
Calories	100	180
Protein	2 G.	6 G.
Carbohydrate	22 G.	28 G.
Fat	1 G.	5 G.

Percentages of U.S. Recommended
Daily Allowances (U.S. RDA)

Protein	2%	10%
Vitamin A	25%	30%
Vitamin C	*	2%
Thiamine	25%	25%
Riboflavin	25%	35%
Niacin	25%	25%
Calcium	*	15%
Iron	25%	25%
Vitamin D	10%	25%
Vitamin B_6	25%	25%
Folic Acid	25%	25%
Vitamin B_{12}	25%	35%
Phosphorus	10%	20%

*Contains less than 2% of the U.S. RDA of these nutrients.

Ingredients: Bran Flakes with other parts of Wheat, Raisins, Sugar, Flavoring, Salt, Honey, Iron, Niacin, Vitamin A, Vitamin B_6, Vitamin B_2, Vitamin B_1, Vitamin D, Folic Acid and Vitamin B_{12}.

Contains 2.5% non-nutritive crude fiber by weight.

As you munch your cereal you can study the package label and learn that by eating one-half cup serving of the product you are getting 35 percent of your RDA of riboflavin and vitamin B_{12}, 30 percent of your requirement of vitamin A, 25 percent of the RDA for thiamine, niacin, iron, vitamin D, vitamin B_6 and folic acid, lesser percentages of your RDA for other vitamins and minerals, six grams of protein, twenty-eight grams of carbohydrate and five grams of fat—in a serving that supplies 180 Calories. You should note that these RDA percentages assume that you put fortified whole milk on your cereal. If for some reason you are eating your cereal dry, assuming you could swallow it, or with skim milk, a number of those percentages would be lower.

The food labeling program is designed to make information on food labels more meaningful to the public. Dr. Alexander M. Schmidt, a former Commissioner of the Food and Drug Administration, has called it "a landmark along the path of modern regulatory initiatives." But the labels won't do any good if you don't read them and take action on the basis of the information given. Of course not all foods carry labels (and you shouldn't expect to see the oranges and grapefruits on your produce shelf disclosing their internal nutritional secrets), but many processed foods now do. So multiply your chances of having a well-balanced meal by dividing your nutrients throughout the day and adding your way to good health.

"BUT I'M A UNIQUE INDIVIDUAL! HOW MUCH AND WHAT SHOULD I EAT?"

Is the Basic Four an adequate guide or does it fail to cover the special requirements of different people?

The answer is simple. A balanced menu built on the Basic Four and variety within each group of the Basic Four, provides for most of us all the constituents necessary for good nutrition. Even if there are special nutrient needs, they are usually met by a well-chosen diet. In the few cases of marked individual differences, what is demanded is generally a reduction of intake rather than an increase. For example, the diabetic decreases the total calories of the diet, not only carbohydrate but also protein and fat; the individual with high blood pressure reduces his intake of sodium. For both the diabetic and hypertensive individual it is *most important* to reduce the total amount of calories and avoid becoming overweight. The individual with high blood cholesterol should cut down on total calories, animal fats, egg yolks, and increase certain vegetable fats to keep the diet palatable and to provide those important polyunsaturates.

In contrast, it is less frequent that an individual will have to add something special to his diet. Individual differences in temporary dietary needs generally arise when an eater has been neglectful of the Basic Four and has adhered to an unbalanced regime. Maybe for that person a correction is necessary. For example: in simple anemia, the requirement for iron is taken care of by frequent consumption of such iron-rich foods as liver, egg yolks, green leafy vegetables, and whole-grain or enriched breads.

Another dietary deficiency—this time a mineral—can be an important cause of dental cavities. Tooth decay caused by lack of fluoride primarily during infancy, childhood and adolescence can be reduced by 60-70 percent if the fluoride content of the public water supply is properly adjusted, a process called "fluoridation." Along the same lines, a moderate increased intake of all the nutrients satisfies the special demands imposed by adolescence, pregnancy, and lactation.

Most of these dietary adjustments are not complicated and can easily be managed. Without question the Basic Four and variety within each group takes care of nearly all the nutritional differences that may exist among individuals, and guides the wise to wise nutrition. It takes the place of the "perfect food" of which there is none.

By far the most common "custom designing" of the Basic Four to meet your own individual needs will focus on the amount of calories you take in and their relationship to your "desirable" weight. You might say this aspect of diet planning is a "matter of form," but it's also a matter of health. So read on to see where you fit on the "underweight" through "obesity" spectrum.

Sizes and Shapes

Size, shape, activity, age and other differences among individuals determine how much is too much, how much is enough. To begin with, a good measure is weight. Do you know what your "desirable weight" is or should be? It is that weight at which the life-insurance companies know you will live the longest. Actually the term "desirable weight" was coined by the Metropolitan Life Insurance Company and is an improvement over a previous term they used: "ideal weight." It is now used by most life-insurance groups and nutrition experts.

A study of thousands of life-insurance records beginning over eighty years ago revealed that those who maintained, for the balance of their lives, the average weight of individuals at age thirty lived longer than the people who gained weight after thirty. At that time (1912) such weights were called "ideal weights."

Further and continuous study of life-insurance records (now in the millions) indicated that the reference age of thirty years was a little high for the best longevity prospects. Average weights at age twenty-five were found to be better, and these were termed "desirable weights."

Desirable weights differ for each sex and are given for three types of body build—small, medium, and large. For men they are higher than for women, and for people with large bones and a big frame they are somewhat more than for those with medium and small body build or frame.

Body build is difficult to determine if one tries to be anthropologically correct. In practice it is simply defined as small, medium, or large. Either you or your physician makes a guess. Glove and shoe sizes are often good guides.

Thus, if you are of medium frame (and most of us are), a female five feet, five inches in height and thirty-two, forty-two, or fifty-two years old, your desirable weight is in the range of 116 to 130 pounds. Desirable weights don't change after the age of twenty-five. Statistics show that women (and men) live longest when they maintain their desirable weight. But we'll get into that more in chapter seven.

Desirable weight is based on weight in average dress. Heights are determined with shoes with two-inch heels. Because the weight figures are for averages only, there is a spread of approximately twelve to fourteen pounds for each level in the table (plus or minus six to seven pounds). This allows for variation in body structure and bone size.

In consulting the table, if you don't know what type frame you have, assume it is medium.

Table 2

WEIGHT IN POUNDS ACCORDING TO FRAME
(In Indoor Clothing)

Desirable weights for men of ages 25 and over

HEIGHT (with shoes on) 1-inch heels	SMALL FRAME	MEDIUM FRAME	LARGE FRAME
5' 2"	112-120	118-129	126-141
5' 3"	115-123	121-133	129-144
5' 4"	118-126	124-136	132-148
5' 5"	121-129	127-139	135-152
5' 6"	124-133	130-143	138-156
5' 7"	128-137	134-147	142-161
5' 8"	132-141	138-152	147-166
5' 9"	136-145	142-156	151-170
5' 10"	140-150	146-160	155-174
5' 11"	144-154	150-165	159-179
6' 0"	148-158	154-170	164-184
6' 1"	152-162	158-175	168-189
6' 2"	156-167	162-180	173-194
6' 3"	160-171	167-185	178-199
6' 4"	164-175	172-190	182-204

Table 3

WEIGHT IN POUNDS ACCORDING TO FRAME
(In Indoor Clothing)

Desirable weights for women of ages 25 and over

HEIGHT (with shoes on) 2-inch heels	SMALL FRAME	MEDIUM FRAME	LARGE FRAME
4' 10"	92- 98	96-107	104-119
4' 11"	94-101	98-110	106-122
5' 0"	96-104	101-113	109-125
5' 1"	99-107	104-116	112-128
5' 2"	102-110	107-119	115-131
5' 3"	105-113	110-122	118-134
5' 4"	108-116	113-126	121-138
5' 5"	111-119	116-130	125-142
5' 6"	114-123	120-135	129-146
5' 7"	118-127	124-139	133-150
5' 8"	122-131	128-143	137-154
5' 9"	126-135	132-147	141-158
5' 10"	130-140	136-151	145-163
5' 11"	134-144	140-155	149-168
6' 0"	138-148	144-159	153-173

For girls between 18 and 25,
subtract 1 pound for each year under 25.

Checking your desirable weight is one part of the weight control formula. The other part is checking how many calories you should be taking in each day to maintain a given weight. Table 4 tells you about that.

Table 4

Daily Calorie Allowance Recommended by Food and
Nutrition Board, National Academy of Sciences—
National Research Council, Revised 1974.

Age	Weight (lbs)	Calories
Males		
11-14	97	2800
15-18	134	3000
19-22	147	3000
23-50	154	2700
51 +	154	2400
Females		
11-14	97	2400
15-18	119	2100
19-22	128	2100
23-50	128	2000
51 +	128	1800
Pregnancy		+300
Lactation		+500

Remember that the column on calories is for total calories throughout a twenty-four-hour period—calories from food and drink from all meals and snacks. If they were just calories from food at our usual three meals, they would be too high. In fact, we think they are too generous for most of us except for those who are pregnant or lactating.

After checking yourself, you may be interested to know how the experts define two words we hear frequently: "overweight" and "obesity," and how they define one word we hear infrequently: "underweight." Overweight means an excess of 10 to 20 percent over desirable body weight. If you boast an excess of 20 percent, you are probably obese. (You might say at that point you had a "Supreme Court Figure"—absolutely no appeal!) On the other hand, if your actual weight is 20 percent or more below your desirable weight, you are underweight.

Suppose your desirable weight is in the 116-130 pound range. If you climb to 140-55, then watch out, you're overweight! If the needle goes on to 160 or above, you are obese, and it's time to stop, look, and go back to the Basic Four *and eat less!* And for those who drink alcoholic beverages, drink less, much less! In the same way, you need a new look and new habits if the pointer drops too low—eat more but don't necessarily drink more.

Be a weight watcher, for your figure's sake and for your health's sake. In planning your meals make sure you give as much consideration to what is on the chairs as you do to what is on the table. Let your scale and the Basic Four be your guides to good nutrition. Only weigh yourself once a week, however, and keep a written record of your weight if it is a problem to you. Daily weighings are meaningless because of fluctuations due to water balance.

We are fortunate that a "fashionable" figure coincides with one that is "desirable" from a very real health point of view.

Nutritious, Delicious and Appealing Too!

Are you well-fed? By that we mean not overfed but wisely fed. Do your meals include all the necessary nutrients?

There is enough food in the United States for everyone. Yet in the midst of abundance, millions are not adequately nourished.

Such inequality is a risky business. In children nutritional deficiency causes poor growth and development; in their elders, the wrong amounts of the wrong foods often result in poor physique, ill health, and even mental grogginess.

One big reason for poor nutrition is waste. Fertile fields are not enough. Our harvest must be intelligently used. Food can be wasted in many ways.

Precious nutrition is lost when foods spoil on pantry shelves or in the refrigerator because of improper purchasing. Often valuable minerals and vitamins are destroyed because foods are overcooked. At other times essential nutrients are poured down the drain when too much cooking water has been used and then most or all of it is discarded.

It makes no sense to squander the vitamins in foods and then hope to make up for this by buying more in a store in the form of pills and powders and supplements of all kinds. Use of dollars for nutritional supplements instead of food is wanton waste.

No nutritional supplement, whatever its claims, contains a short-cut to health. There is no miracle food and no magic in any special dietary regimen. Many different foods and many different patterns of eating can all lead to good nutrition.

The "Basic Four"—dairy products; enriched and whole-grain breads and cereals; fruits and vegetables; meat, eggs, fish, and poultry—provide a generous amount of health-building nutrients. All of these are plentiful in the United States. If you purchase them properly and use them wisely, you *will* be well-fed.

But nutrients aren't enough. Meals must not only be good; they must *look* good too. There is one resolution a housewife can make any day of the year and that is to keep her family's meals attractive as well as wholesome.

It is especially important to have a cheerful table in the winter when days are dreary and spirits sag. All through the year, however, the amount of consumption is increased and waste and leftovers decreased if food is tempting and tasty.

There are three keys to eye and taste appeal: color, texture, and flavor.

Consider color. Could anything be less appetizing than an all-white meal of baked fish, mashed potatoes, and creamed cauliflower? What a difference color could make—paprika and lemon slices on the fish; cheese in the white sauce; and a garnish of green parsley! Brightened with color accents, any food looks and even tastes better.

Interesting texture helps too. In that imaginary fish-and-potato meal everything is soft. Crisp it up with a tossed vegetable salad or with some carrot and celery sticks, and the whole effect is changed.

Variety Is The Spice of Life!

Variations in flavor are vital too. Monotony vanishes when something new is added to a weary old dish. The number of herbs, spices, and seasonings available is great, their uses unending. For example, the addition of oregano makes for a change in soup or salad dressing; or that of bay leaf in the water when potatoes are boiled for mashing. Thyme adds a new touch to green beans and scallions pep up peas.

Meals perk up when you keep a file of favorite menus and a list of new and different recipes. Then, even in a jiffy, mouth-watering meals can come from frozen, canned, and prepared food.

Even a quick company meal can amaze the guests. Such a menu might be: a canned or packaged, dried French onion soup sprinkled with grated Parmesan cheese; canned ham that has an orange-marmalade glacé; canned sweet potatoes, placed in a buttered baking dish on thinly sliced lemon, sprinkled with a little sugar and salt, and seasoned with a few cloves and a stick of cinnamon; a canned green vegetable; and, to top it all off, a dessert of canned peach halves brushed with butter or margarine, filled with canned mincemeat, and popped into the broiler for a few minutes. The dinner is easy; it's full of vitamins and minerals; and it has originality in color and texture and flavor.

Good planning can make all the difference in nutrition and in satisfaction! Be bold; try new combinations. Keep variety in mind. And keep up with the variation of fresh fruits and vegetables you'll find in your grocery produce section as the seasons change. Have you ever heard of a salad made with a base of a pineapple ring on top of some lettuce, cottage cheese in the hole in the pineapple, and the whole thing covered over with some cold canned sauerkraut? It's good.

And you should vary your meats too. Burgers, poultry, veal and pork are great, but when you deserve a break, remember such items as liver, kidney, heart, sweetbreads, brains, tongue, and tripe. Gourmets are wild about them. European chefs have built reputations upon them. Families abroad consider them palate-tantalizing delicacies.

But not in the United States.

An occasional restaurant makes a specialty of one or more of the variety meats, but the appeal is selective rather than popular.

The variety meats should have a high place on the thrifty housewife's shopping list. The fact that they don't may at least be due partly to the fact that she is unfamiliar with them and with the methods of preparing them.

Variety meats can be recommended on several counts. They are high in nutrition, with protein, iron, and the B-complex vitamins (thiamine, riboflavin, niacin).

With all these advantages, you can add one more: they are the least expensive cuts of meat, a real economy food with all the nutritional benefits.

Just as the name implies, there are a variety of ways of preparing these meats. Liver is the best known of the group. It is most frequently served braised with onions or bacon. It can be equally delectable ground and used in a liver loaf, liver patties or as sandwich spread. And how about a liver chow mein or a casserole?

Excellent dishes can also be prepared with the other variety meats. Steak-and-kidney pie is a delicacy with the British. Sweetbreads are considered a party-fare favorite. They are tasty as appetizers or served en brochette. Baked stuffed heart is known the world over.

Tongue can be roasted, boiled, smoked or pickled. It is wonderful as a main dish or in sandwiches.

Tripe, part of the stomach of animals, has been grossly and unfairly libeled throughout the centuries. The word itself has come to mean anything bad or worthless. But nutritionally, it is a food far from worthless. Any good cookbook has numerous recipes for preparing it. So be brave! Experiment with new dishes!

And speaking of experimenting—and diversifying menus—with variety meat, keep in mind that there are many ways of eating for good health, all within the Basic Four, but spread among the dishes of many cultures.

Whether it is pumpkin pie or Chinese fried rice, much of our food has a special history, and we are richer for it. Protein is necessary for all of us. If our heritage is Mexican-American we can get a healthy amount of it at a low cost from such traditional dishes as refried beans. One of the many delicious so-called "Jewish foods," chopped chicken livers, is an excellent source of iron. And if you decide to experiment with soul food, you may find yourself fixing grits and turnip greens and when you do you are serving up portions of iron, vitamin A, B vitamins and vitamin C. So be an international gourmet a la the Basic Four.

Elegant and Nutritious Are Not Contradictory

Speaking of gourmet dishes, you should always remember that gourmet food can be glamourous *and* nutritious too. A proper diet can give your entire family real enjoyment and ensure good health— including good heart health. Just for example, consider a menu of Chicken Imperial, a chicken simmered in a delicious wine sauce (you'll find the recipe for this in the Appendix with others designed to give your heart a break) and garnished with small baby onions and a cup of freshly sliced mushrooms. Sound elegant? It is, but then chicken is an inexpensive, excellent, low-fat, low-cholesterol source of protein of excellent nutritional quality. Just dress it up a bit and it becomes special.

In planning your elegant evenings, keep in mind also that protein foods need not be limited to the main course. Your dinner can take on a real flare if occasionally you serve a nutritious appetizer such as marinated herring, shrimp cocktail or crab meat—or a good hearty soup. You can even "sneak" proteins into desserts—fruit whips made with egg whites are a good source, as well as puddings made with milk. Desserts may be made with skim milk which contains as much protein but only half as many calories as whole milk and almost no fat. This can be a boon to the weight watcher or to anyone on a low-fat diet.

THREE MEALS A DAY—PLUS SENSIBLE SNACKING

You can be sure of good foods and good meals if you have a variety of foods and three regular meals. Why?

Because morning, noon, and night one should have about one-fifth to one-third of a day's food needs. This assures a good supply of nutrients and permits room for snacks for pleasure and efficiency in the hours between meals. People who always rely on doughnuts and coffee, or similar snacks, end up by cheating themselves of the nutrients necessary for optimum health and vigor. Have variety in snacks as well.

Meals and snacks can be flexible in all sorts of ways, but during each twenty-four hours they should include all the Basic Four foods.

Briefly, this means that every day each person should have: (1) two servings of meat, fish, poultry or cheese; (2) two servings of fruit and two servings of vegetables, and (3) several servings of whole-grain or enriched bread or cereal. And here we repeat again, adjust the size of the servings to your body weight. In addition, adults should have one or two glasses of milk, or some cheese. Rapidly growing children and pregnant and lactating women should have more.

All this can be done easily, with the following model meal plan:

BREAKFAST

Fruit or juice. This is a good time to make sure of vitamin C (with citrus fruit or other juice fortified with added vitamin C).

Protein food. Cereal with milk, cheese, or even hamburger if you prefer. Don't feel inhibited by tradition!

Energy food. Toast or roll. Spread: margarine or jam.

Beverage.

MAIN MEAL (whether at noon or night)

Protein. Three to four ounces of meat, fish or poultry.

Energy food. Potato, rice, macaroni, noodles or bread, or a combination.

Vegetable. This can be cooked or raw, or you can have both.

Fruit, or other dessert.

Beverage.

LUNCH OR SUPPER

Protein. Cheese or slice of meat or poultry or small portion of fish.

Vegetable.

Energy food. Similar to main meal choices. Spread: margarine.

Fruit.

Beverage.

This pattern can be tailored by each person according to age and activity, weight and waistline. So look at the scale, look at yourself, and then decide: (1) how big the portions should be; (2) the amount of fat you require; (3) the amount of bread and spread you should use; (4) the type of dessert that is best for you; (5) how much sugar and other sweets you need; (6) the kind of beverage you should have; (7) how many snacks and extras you can allow yourself; and (8) how many and what kind of alcoholic beverages, if any!

If you follow these simple suggestions, you have an A-1 meal plan! It has balance and variety for good and healthful eating. And forget the Tiger's Milk, wheat germ, and other nutritional supplements.

A Good Breakfast Is a Good Idea!

A good breakfast is good for you. This is more than just a slogan, and for old or young it is true. And because this is the one of the three meals that most often gets "cheated" in favor of frenzied morning activity, or simply a few moments extra in bed, it's worth discussing in some detail.

Carefully designed research projects, studies of every sort, have proved that there are sound scientific reasons for a "good" breakfast.

The most evident reason for eating breakfast is literally to "break your fast." For most of us it has been ten to twelve hours since we last ate.

There is another good reason for having breakfast. Without this first meal it is difficult to obtain the day's quota of essential nutrients. Studies show that children who do not eat breakfast invariably have a less desirable food intake than those who eat a regular morning meal. Among all groups, especially adolescents, non-breakfast eaters have the most inadequate nutrition records.

Usually youngsters themselves are not to blame. They lack the judgment necessary for wise meal planning. Parents have the responsibility of preparing an interesting breakfast and of seeing that it is eaten without fuss or commotion. Both parents need to set a good example and not to make breakfast a hurried swallow of coffee followed by a quick cigarette.

For every member of the family, lack of breakfast makes a poor start for the day. Work output suffers at home, at school, and at the office or on the job.

Youngsters who have not eaten in the morning are very often the ones who do not do well at school. They are restless and inattentive; they tire easily and have little energy for outdoor activity.

Adolescents and young adults show similar reactions. Research was done on this group a number of years ago at the University of Iowa. Reaction time, maximum work output, and neuromuscular tremor were measured after there had been: (1) no breakfast; (2) only black coffee; (3) moderate breakfast; and (4) heavy breakfast. In nearly all cases no breakfast had an unfavorable effect. Black coffee alone proved to be even more detrimental. Heavy breakfast resulted in a decrease in work output for adults but not for adolescents. A moderate, good breakfast was best for most.

What *is* a good breakfast? Anything you like as long as it supplies about one-fourth of the daily requirements for calories, protein, and other necessary constituents. Good protein has two important effects. First, it prevents a feeling of pre-lunchtime hunger and weakness. Second, experimental work has suggested that the presence of some protein food in a meal increases the body's utilization of other essential nutrients.

If the traditional breakfast foods are dull or unappetizing to you or your child, there is no reason why you have to eat them. A hamburger on a bun or a grilled cheese sandwich is just as nutritious in the morning as at noon. One youngster we know will eat a fresh-fruit sundae with great relish for breakfast but won't look at milk or plain fruit. For most of us, though, a delicious and tantalizing meal can be based on the traditional breakfast foods: fruit, milk or coffee or tea, toast, jam, cereal, ham or bacon.

A good breakfast gives a head start on the day's work and on its nutritional needs. Those who claim they "can't face food in the morning and never eat breakfast" are neglecting their health and disregarding the expectations of their families, their employers, their teachers, and themselves.

And speaking of teachers, schools play an important role in the proper nutrition of our youngsters. A good breakfast will get them through the morning. A good lunch helps keep them bright all afternoon. Read about the all-importance of nutritious school lunch programs in chapter six.

Nibble Knowledgably!

Snacks and nibbles can be *good* habits. This is possible, that is, if we plan on them and they are pleasant! Eating between meals is a pretty well-established custom, especially for children. Unfortunately, snacking does not always improve the nutritional qualities of a poor diet.

It is estimated that as much as 10 to 20 percent of a person's calorie needs are supplied by nibbles. This is of considerable importance, particularly for weight watchers and for youngsters.

Poorly planned and unevenly spaced meals often cause the amount of between-meal eating to be increased. However, if done properly, snacking can be put to good use. Sensible snacks, properly timed, can help allay fatigue and emotional upsets in young children. Some youngsters simply cannot eat all they need in three meals. Four or five small meals a day that are eaten will be more likely to provide the essentials of good nutrition than two or three large ones that are only partially eaten. *Good food supplies good nutrition only when it is consumed!*

For the person who needs to gain weight, snacks and nibbles may help solve the problem. Extra calories can be sneaked in without interfering with mealtimes. In this case it is important to space the snacks so they are not too close to mealtime. They should come nearer to the last meal rather than to the next meal. Also, a fairly substantial bedtime snack can help put on the necessary pounds.

Even if you weigh too much, you can have snacks. Some people find it easier to stay on a reduced calorie intake if the pattern is planned to include between-meal and bedtime snacks. They help control hunger and provide the satisfaction one gets from eating. These nibbles must be part of your diet. They should come shortly before a meal to dull your appetite. They are not something extra taken in addition to a meal but really a part of the meal simply eaten earlier.

Good foods for snacks are ones that add to the essential nutrient value of the diet. They are planned for and are a part of your diet. We like to think of them as "scientific" nibbles, in contrast to "common" ones. Common nibbles are extras. They are in addition to your regular diet. A good rule is to choose your snacks from the "Basic Four" food groups and from the foods you would ordinarily consume at mealtime. Then you can be sure they are "scientific."

If you like, eat snacks and enjoy them. They play an important part in our social as well as our nutritional customs. Just be aware of them. Examine your snack habits. Are they the proper ones for you? Nutritious snacks include: nuts, cheese and crackers, a glass of milk, ice cream, potato or corn chips, cookies—and with these foods a soft drink or glass of beer to give zest and enjoyment to snack time.

And don't forget about soup! Millions of Americans eat soup for lunch and dinner—some even for breakfast! Soup is popular the world around. In fact, "Soup's on" has become almost synonymous with, "Come and get it," or, in good party-manner lingo, "Dinner is served." And it's also great for snack time.

Soup is good, and it's good for you. It fits well in everyone's diet, no matter what his age. Like any other food, particularly those that are liquid, when consumed in excess, they fill you up. Then other nutritious foods are not consumed, and one may have an unbalanced diet. This is especially true with preschool-age children with fickle appetites.

Children usually love soup, and that's a good thing. Mothers love soup too. Busy mothers, in particular, enjoy the convenience of prepared soups. They're so easy to fix in the midst of a hectic day. Just open the container and, if called for, mix with water or milk. The soups definitely taste "uncanny!"

Poor food habits may be formed, not by the fact that children eat soup, but because they sometimes eat too much of it—too much because they pass up the meat, vegetables, and fruits they need to balance their diets. So watch that too.

THOSE SEASONAL SPLURGES

The special occasions in our life need special attention. Holidays like Easter, Passover, Thanksgiving, Christmas and Hanukkah. And don't forget the festivities that go with summer too! You can still enjoy—even budget an occasional splurge, but you still do have to count calories and make sure you're within the all-year-round Basic Four.

Eat, Drink and Be Merry—Moderately!

Holiday meals can be pleasant and painless if you don't panic. If you and your family exercise a little care (and your muscles as well!) you can have your cake and eat it too (unless it's *very, very* rich and fancy!).

It won't be possible to cram too many festive foods into too many meals at holiday time, but if the goodies are spread out evenly and sensibly you can definitely retain your trim waistline and the flavor of the season as well.

Remember, you do not become overweight between Christmas and New Year's, but between New Year's and Christmas. Almost always what causes obesity is eating a little too much day after day, week after week over a long period of time, and not burning up those extra calories in extra physical activities. If you have good eating habits, and good exercise habits, then the special occasions are not fatal, and you can even indulge in a holiday bonus here and there.

Holiday foods aren't necessarily higher in calories than those we eat every day. Some are higher, it's true: candied sweet potatoes have about 200 more calories than mashed potatoes; turkey stuffing may add calories. Chiefly, however, it is the extras that count, the extra times and the extra foods, without the extra physical activity, that make not sense but excess.

Life can't be day after day of meticulous calorie budgeting, but it's worthwhile to think and plan before you splurge! You know there is such a thing as splurging wisely. The bathroom scale is the final judge of your wisdom.

Being Thankful—Or Just Plain Full?

Thanksgiving Day is a useful example of where we can celebrate wisely. Let's get up to date! What was good for the Pilgrims isn't necessarily good for us. The rugged ways of Colonial times are gone forever. Menus made in 1600 are equally outdated today.

Way back in the seventeenth century the newly arrived colonists barely survived their first winter in Plymouth, Massachusetts. Nearly half of them died of disease, exposure and starvation. You may recall, however, that food crops during the next summer were so bountiful that Governor William Bradford decreed December 13, 1621, to be a day of feasting and prayer. The colonists—men, women and children—worked for weeks toward the celebration. Turkey, deer, geese, ducks and fish were caught by the men. The women prepared vegetables, fruits and accompaniments. It was a great undertaking for all.

When the Pilgrims sat down to a groaning holiday table they had hunted their own turkeys, grown their own vegetables. They had ground their own meal, lugged their water from a well, chopped and hauled wood for their fires. They needed abundant calories after all these activities.

By contrast, think of today's Thanksgiving! Foods come from supermarket shelves; mechanical wonders do the cooking and transportation. After dinner's done, most everyone sits down to watch football on TV.

No doubt about it, the seventies are sedentary. Pounds piled on at a Thanksgiving feast aren't exercised away. Ten pounds this year may become more pounds next year and another new waist measure the year after that. The increased waistline means a decreased lifeline; obesity is perhaps the greatest of all health hazards in the United States today.

We just cannot use the extra calories that were essential for the Pilgrims three hundred years ago, so let's enjoy an up-to-date Thanksgiving dinner. The modern way is the moderate way.

Fortunately, turkey is still a fine tradition. It's low in fat and provides the polyunsaturated fatty acids that are beneficial. Furthermore, turkey's a good source of protein and also supplies minerals and vitamins. Vegetables, too, are always healthful. Even the starchiest don't add too much to the calorie scale if they are cooked carefully and not adorned with rich sauces or fat.

Then where are the calories?

First of all, there's a hazard in the snacks that accompany the festive drinks or first course. Maybe they're small, but they're rich. So keep the count down. Or better still, nibble on raw vegetables and save space for what's to follow. Don't forget, the drinks have calories too—more in martinis, less in cranberry juice.

Stuffing's another storehouse of calories. It's a good idea in preparation to use more celery and onion and somewhat less bread and to moisten with broth instead of fat. Then, remember, don't eat too much!

Make twentieth-century gravy, too. Use the refrigerator to cool the juices; then skim off the fat, add broth or water from cooked vegetables, and thicken with a little flour. That's a gravy that's full of flavor, full of good nutrition, and fine for the figure too!

Finally, since there's such an abundance of foods, keep all the portions small. Slim down that slice of pie. Praise the hostess, but save the seconds for another day.

Grim? No—you can still enjoy. Wise? Yes. For better health throughout the year use a large measure for your thanks, but a small measure for your servings.

The advice about eating at Thanksgiving is applicable to other holidays as well. Consider some of the typical holiday and everyday foods listed below by their caloric value. Compare your own holiday fare with your own everyday meals, and you'll probably find similar differences in the caloric "bottom line."

HOLIDAY FOODS

	Calories
Ham, 3½ ounces	397
Duck or goose, roasted, 3 slices	315
Turkey, roasted, 3 slices	200
Bread stuffing, ½ cup	233
Cranberry jelly, 1 rounded tablespoon	47
Candied sweet potatoes, 2 halves	358
Fruit cake	142
Mince pie	398
Hard sauce, 2 tablespoons	100
English walnuts, 8 to 15 halves	100
Eggnog, Christmas type, 1 punch cup	335

EVERYDAY FOODS

Hamburger, 3½ ounces	236
Meat loaf, 3½ ounces	377
Mashed potatoes, ½ cup	123
French-fried potatoes, 10 strips	200
Bread, 1 slice	63
Apple pie	377
Chocolate cupcake with fudge icing	278
Brownie	141
Jelly doughnut	226
Chocolate ice-cream soda	255

You need not despair or spoil the epicurean delights of holiday foods. Eating is meant to be one of the pleasures of life, and this menu shows how you can have the traditional joys—for only 1900 Calories.

BREAKFAST

Broiled grapefruit half
Cereal and milk
Toast—1 slice
Jelly—1 teaspoon
Beverage

COCKTAIL HOUR

Vegetable juice, or soft drink
Highball—one
Shrimp with cocktail sauce

DINNER

Sliced breast of roast young tom turkey—3 to 4 ounces
Southern cornbread stuffing—1/3 cup
Giblet gravy—2 tablespoons
Fresh broccoli with lemon—1 serving
Holiday apple-grape salad—1 serving
Cranberry sherbet
Beverage

SUPPER

Cold sliced turkey—3 ounces
Cranberry sauce
Dinner roll and butter
Stuffed celery hearts and olives
Orange ambrosia (flavored with Kirsch)
Beverage

The idea is to attack the holiday table with prudence. Think "stuffed" when sitting down to the table. Take small portions—and keep up a strong willpower when seconds are passed. If visiting and your hostess serves with a generous hand, adopt the old English custom of leaving at least one-fourth of each food portion on your plate for the "poor." In Merry Old England, food left on the plate was a method of charity as the uneaten was literally doled out to the poor. Our purpose isn't the same, but equally important as our bodies benefit.

Exercise is the order for this day as all the rest—maybe more so. Fancy, calorie-laden recipes are brought out for this day. So if jogging is your practice, make sure it's on the gobbler-day schedule. If not, long walks and/or other exercise are worth our time investment.

And there is advice for the cook—compose foods with consideration of calories. Keep it simple! Bring flavor to the meal with combinations of seasonings, spices and herbs and keep a frugal hand on margarine or butter and other calorie-loaded ingredients. Calories always count—holiday or no holiday.

Food Sense for Summer

When summer comes around, with its temptations for over- or underindulging in food and drink, don't let the weather side-track you and your family into poor food habits.

Regardless of the temperature, you still need calories, protein, minerals, and vitamins. When the weather is hot, most of us need fewer calories than in the winter, chiefly because we do less physically. But we still need well-planned meals of food chosen wisely for variety and for balance.

The temptation to "cool off" with iced drinks, Popsicles, and ices is great. These furnish calories, maybe more than you need, and they can also spoil your appetite for planned meals.

Picnics, cookouts, and the call of the open spaces can be hard on middle-aged or older people and may lead to eating and exercising too much at one time.

Also, remember that beer, gin and tonic, and rum collins all furnish calories. A "drink" before dinner should mean no dessert if you want to keep from gaining, or, hopefully, remove a pound or two.

So why not be careful and wise! Take advantage of the heat and the wonderful supply of summer foods to plan meals that will help the weight watchers, and will also be lower in fat than most of our usual ones. Many doctors feel that regulating calories to reach and maintain "desirable weight" is of practical value as a health measure.

The following menu is an example. It furnishes only about 1850 Calories (300-400 less than most of us usually consume), and it has only about two-thirds as much fat as the usual American menu (32-34 percent of the calories from fat versus 40 percent). We recommend it, and variations, for good, well-balanced summertime nutrition.

BREAKFAST

½ medium cantaloupe or serving of berries
cereal and milk
1 slice toast
1 pat margarine
1 glass of milk
Coffee or tea (no cream)

MID-MORNING

1 glass chilled fruit juice and soda water (half and half)

NOON

Jellied consomme with lemon slice
Melba toast
Crabmeat salad on lettuce with tomato quarters, 1 tbsp. salad dressing
Pineapple sherbet
Cookie
Iced tea (with lemon and sugar, if desired)

MID-AFTERNOON

Iced tea, lemon or limeade, or Coke

DINNER

Tomato-juice cocktail
Roast chicken (no gravy)
Parsley new potatoes
1 pat margarine
Fresh peas and new onions with mint
Fresh fruit salad on lettuce (no dressing)
Lemon meringue pie
Iced coffee (no cream)

BEDTIME

Chilled buttermilk or beer
Saltines

TREATING YOUR TEETH TO GOOD NUTRITION

Good teeth are a precious possession. We have to have them for an attractive smile, for enjoyment of daily meals, for good digestion.

Bright, white teeth may look as solid as the rock of Gilbraltar, but appearances are sadly deceiving. Ask anyone who has lived through an hour—or five minutes—of a toothache, or of a dentist's drill. Ask anyone who has seen older people existing on pureed pap because of neglected teeth. Elimination of such miseries is a goal worth everyone's attention.

One vital need is to build better teeth with the right foods at the right time. Proper dental care means not only good hygiene but also good nutrition all through life.

The good nutrition has to start at the very beginning. So a must for mothers during pregnancy is a well-balanced diet. After birth there must be a supply of tooth-building nutrients for the second teeth as they begin to grow. Once they have appeared, they need the best possible lifetime care to keep them in good working condition.

For a long time it has been recognized that tooth enamel and dentin require the minerals calcium and phosphorus, protein, and the vitamins A and D, and that gums cannot be healthy without vitamin C. More recently, studies conducted for more than a generation have shown that without any question very small amounts of fluoride greatly decrease the amount of dental decay—by 60 to 70 percent.

Every individual from his first day on must have the foods that provide tooth-building minerals and vitamins: milk and cheese, citrus fruits, green and yellow vegetables, and enriched or whole-grain bread and cereal.

Probably one of the most important threats your teeth face is that of dental caries—that is, cavities. Dental caries today is probably the most prevalent chronic disease afflicting man and particularly in areas where the water supply does not have the right amount of fluoride—about 1 to 1.2 milligrams per quart of water. This is usually referred to as 1 ppm (one part fluoride per million parts of water).

Why do these caries develop? Some people, particularly food faddists and the so-called consumer activists, are quick to blame white, refined sugar (naturally, brown sugar and honey are OK!) for all dental problems. But the situation is, of course, more complex than that. The fact remains that the risk of dental caries is increased when sugar products are consumed *between* meals, particularly in sticky form so it adheres to the teeth. But sugar consumed with meals is no more conducive to tooth decay than any other type of carbohydrate.

Fluoridation: The Lowest Price Insurance You Can Buy!

By far the most important thing you can do to protect the teeth of your children and grandchildren from tooth decay is to see that your community has the intelligence to adjust the fluoride content of its water. This is called "fluoridation." Fluoridation currently and for the forseeable future is the most effective, economic and practical means of preventing dental caries. This single step alone, when fluoridated water is consumed from infancy on, will reduce dental decay by 60 to 70 percent, and fluoridation of public water supplies only costs about fifty cents per person per year (yes, per year, not per day). This favorable effect is permanent as long as one continues to drink fluoridated water. That is a pretty good bargain in the field of public health.

Fluoridation has its opponents, just as every important step in public health has had—vaccination against smallpox and iodization of salt, to name a couple. One of the favorite arguments against the procedure is that fluoride is a poison. This is true: it is—in large amounts. But the amount present in water, naturally or by addition, is so small that it makes this argument ridiculous. Many of the things we use or eat every day can be "poisonous" in large amounts. Chlorine, used for purifying water, is toxic if used in large amounts. So are vitamins A and D; so even are such common substances as salt and water; in fact, so is everything if taken in large enough quantities.

You'll hear fluoridation opponents complain about the possibility that individuals are allergic to fluoride. But the American Academy of Allergy has repeatedly evaluated this question and concluded: "There is no evidence of allergy or intolerance to fluorides as used in the fluoridation of community water supplies." What more proof would you want?

But the arguments go on. Some antifluoridationists, in their desperate and varied attempts to delay further adoption of one of the greatest advances in modern public health, drag in the issue of pollution. Their question usually is "why pollute our waters further by adding this dangerous chemical fluoride?" The fact remains, of course, that fluoridation in no way contributes to any pollution problem. As summarized by Nobel Laureate Dr. Albert Szent-Gyorgyi, "I think fluoridation is one of the major advances in preventive medicine. I [would have been] spared a great deal of trouble and have had a smoother life had I had fluoridated water in my youth. Fluoride is a natural constituent of our surroundings and it is chiefly due to man's emancipation of nature that we do not get enough of it. Dental caries is one of the major annoyances of life which do not always stop at the annoyance level but can seriously threaten life and happiness."

If you are faced with the responsibility of deciding whether your city fluoridates its water supply, don't be frightened by the scare tactics of fluoridation's emotional opponents. Many millions of people have lived for centuries in areas where fluoride exists naturally in their water supply. You will have nothing to lose and much to gain from fluoridation. Today over 100 million people in over 5,000 communities enjoy the health benefits of fluoridation, and this includes almost all of our major cities. In these areas tooth decay is decreasing.

Is *your* area fluoridated? Check your city's fluoridation status on the list we've included. If your city is not listed there—and you're not living in one of those states with laws requiring fluoridation, call your health department and ask them. If your water is not fluoridated, get involved in community health activities and let your health department know that you want fluoridation. If it becomes necessary to have a referendum on the matter, help get out a big "yes" vote.

Fluoridation Status of Biggest U. S. Cities*

Dates indicate initiation of fluoridation

Population one million and over		Population 250,000 – 499,999	
New York	1965	Atlanta	1969
Chicago	1956	Buffalo	1955
Los Angeles	no	Cincinnati	1976
Philadelphia	1954	Nashville	1953
Detroit	1967	Minneapolis	1957
		Fort Worth	1965
		Toledo	1955
Population 500,000 – 999,999		Portland	no
		Newark	no
		Oklahoma City	1954
Baltimore	1952	Oakland	1976
Dallas	1966	Louisville	1951
Washington, D.C.	1952	Long Beach	1971
Cleveland	1956	Omaha	1969
Indianapolis	1951	Tulsa	1953
Milwaukee	1953	Miami	1952
San Francisco	1952	Honolulu	no
San Diego	no	St. Paul	1952
San Antonio	no	Norfolk	1952
Boston	1978	Birmingham	no
Memphis	1970	Rochester, NY	1952
St. Louis	1955	Tampa	no
New Orleans	1974	Wichita	no
Phoenix	no	Akron	1969
Columbus, Ohio	1973	Tucson	no
Seattle	1969	Jersey City	1974
Pittsburgh	1952	Sacramento	no
Denver	1954	Austin	1973
Kansas City, MO	no	Richmond	1952

States With Laws Requiring Fluoridation

Connecticut	1965	Michigan	1968
Minnesota	1967	South Dakota	1969
Illinois	1967	Ohio	1969
Kentucky	1976	Georgia	1973
		Nebraska	1973

*From U.S. Public Health Service, "Fluoridation 1975."

How does your state stand on fluoridation?* The first number for each state refers to the percentage of its population on public water supplied with natural or controlled fluoridation. The second number shows the state's population in a ranking of all states according to percentages.

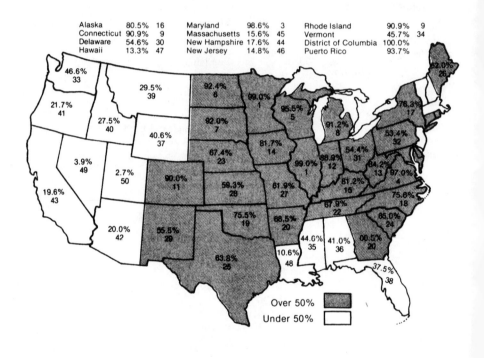

Alaska	80.5%	16	Maryland	98.6%	3	Rhode Island	90.9%	9
Connecticut	90.9%	9	Massachusetts	15.6%	45	Vermont	45.7%	34
Delaware	54.6%	30	New Hampshire	17.6%	44	District of Columbia	100.0%	
Hawaii	13.3%	47	New Jersey	14.8%	46	Puerto Rico	93.7%	

Over 50% ▓
Under 50% ☐

*Map used with permission of *Nutrition Today*.

You'll hear the argument that goes "fluoride only benefits children so I don't want it in my water." But the people who make this statement are not only selfish but not keeping up with scientific knowledge about the broader health implications of fluorides in the diet.

Studies over a decade have shown that the mineral nutrient fluoride has a beneficial effect in the treatment and prevention of diseases having nothing to do with tooth decay, namely osteoporosis and possibly in calcification of the vascular tissues, probably better known to you as hardening of the arteries.

Osteoporosis, the most commonly seen metabolic bone disease in adults, particularly those beyond the mid-fifties, literally means porous bones. In this disease the bones lose calcium, and they become less "calcified." Frequently the vertebrae, the bones in the spinal column, collapse, causing back pain. A few doctors have recently used large amounts of fluoride to treat this disease with gratifying results in many individuals; the bones become better calcified and less likely to fracture, and the patients have less pain. The amounts of fluoride used for this purpose are far larger than obtained from fluoridated water.

Because of these observations, researchers at Harvard's Department of Nutrition decided to see if there would be less osteoporosis in adults over forty-five years of age who lived for a long period of time in areas where the drinking water contained high amounts of fluoride (4.0 to 5.8 parts per million or four to six times more fluoride than customarily added to city water supplies lacking this nutrient) than in those living in areas with small amounts of fluoride (0.15 to 0.30 parts per million).

They found that there was much less osteoporosis among adults in the high fluoride area than in the low fluoride area. They also had a much lower incidence of collapsed vertebrae and fewer complaints of back pain than persons living in the low fluoride areas. Another exciting finding was that X-rays showed much less calcification (hardening) of the aorta (the major blood vessel leaving the heart) in the adults living in the high fluoride area.

Thus, the mineral nutrient fluoride not only helps protect the teeth from decay, but reduces the incidence of osteoporosis and may lessen or slow down hardening of the arteries. The mineral nutrient fluoride apparently helps to keep calcium in the hard tissues of the body (teeth and bones) and out of the soft tissues such as the aorta and other blood vessels.

We've presented some of the basic principles of good health and tips for applying these basics to everyday eating. But meal planning and general nutritional decision-making in the mid and late 1970s may lead to some additional questions. So let's take a look at them.

Chapter Four
Eating and Drinking in a Modern World

Our lives today are really very complex. Literally dozens of different activities are competing for our time. Where a century ago most people grew their own vegetables and raised their own cattle and poultry or purchased it directly from a farm in the neighborhood, today the overwhelming majority of us rely on modern food technology and the local grocery or supermarket for the food we eat. We expect a large variety of fresh, nutritious, attractive food to be readily available to us. And at fair prices!

The next time you are wheeling your shopping cart up and down the long aisles of your food market stop for a moment and consider the variety—and yes, quality—of the food we have, compared to those of past generations. Because of sophisticated screening measures, we don't have to worry about the safety of the food on our shelves. In earlier days, food safety was a real source of concern. We are not significantly affected by major weather changes that could affect produce availability. Of course there are fluctuations in the cost of fresh produce by season and availability, but we have a large assortment of canned, frozen and other processed foods to select from all year round.

Eating in a modern world has its definite advantages. But it has raised some concerns too. In many ways, food science is moving ahead faster than public awareness about its progress. And in the midst of our current "food revolution" some consumers, perhaps you too, have become confused. Again, the questions being raised about the "goodness" of modern foods provide the perfect setting for food faddist fare. One of the entrepreneurial areas faddists have had the most success in recent years is that of vitamin supplements. Let's take a closer look at that topic.

EAT, DRINK AND SUPPLEMENT!??

Is this the rule we should follow?

If you are eating a well-balanced diet and your physician has not prescribed a nutrient supplement for you, the answer is "no." But that answer is so important, it's worth elaborating upon.

We are surrounded by claims of the wonders of so-called "natural" vitamins, and more recently, megavitamins. The next time you see such an advertisement, beware. A vitamin is a vitamin. There is nothing richer about the ones that have the label "natural," except perhaps the individual who is selling them to you. And "natural" or otherwise, you are not accomplishing anything by taking vitamin supplements; indeed you may in certain cases be threatening your health and certainly you are unnecessarily depleting your food budget. Those "high-potency" vitamins, or megavitamins, can be expensive! So can the elaborate "health juicers" which boast of being able to extract the natural vitality from organically-grown garden goodies. But let's get vitamin-specific.

Vitamin A

Are you taking vitamin A or eating inordinate amounts of foods which have carotene, the substance from which our bodies make vitamin A? Before you take your next dose, keep these facts in mind: excess intake of vitamin A can create havoc to your health.

Most foods that occur in nature do not have enough vitamin A to bring about problems. But in 1856 an arctic explorer documented an exception to that rule. He and his companions feasted one night on a healthy serving of polar bear liver, and, shortly after, recorded symptoms of dizziness, violent frontal headache and nausea, drowsiness and irritability. A century later, diners enjoying shark liver reported the same effects. Both groups had eaten food which contained an extraordinary amount of vitamin A, and they were experiencing its toxic effects.

Today very few of us include polar bear or fish livers in our diet, but on the other hand, many well-meaning consumers are taking high supplementary doses of vitamin A. And physicians are reporting side effects. Of particular concern is the observation that those suffering from vitamin A intoxication report the same type of intracranial pressure and violent headaches that are associated with brain tumors. More than once a serious and unnecessary operation has been performed.

Do you want some more evidence on why you shouldn't overdo the vitamin intake? One woman who purchased her $250 "juicer" and $42 blender from her health-food store and drank over a quart of carrot and other vegetable juice daily, noted that the bottoms of her feet and palms of her hands became yellow. When she explained her problem to the owner of her health-food store he responded, "Good, the impurities of your liver are being cleansed, and they are working themselves out through your skin." Actually, however, this woman and many like her developed a disease known as carotenemia, due to the excessive consumption of the yellow pigment, carotene.

But wait, there's more. *The New York Times* recently carried the story of a forty-eight-year-old health-food enthusiast who, according to a coroner's inquest, had died from "carrot juice addiction." The individual in question had taken 70 million IU of vitamin A over a period of ten days and, in addition, was drinking about a gallon of carrot juice during that time. His skin was bright yellow when he died. The effect of the enormous intake of vitamin A from the carrots and vitamin tablets was indistinguishable from alcoholic poisoning of the liver. It produced the same result—cirrhosis of the liver.

So how can you make sure you don't abuse vitamin A? First, you can avoid the temptation to take vitamin A capsules—unless, of course, your physician prescribes them for a specific need. Second, you can eat a well-balanced diet, forget about blenders and fancy devices and chew your carrots and other vegetables the way the rest of us do. If you are eating normal quantities of foods and passing up supplements you have absolutely no reason to be concerned about overdosing yourself with vitamin A.

As with the case of vitamin A, you can do yourself harm by taking too much vitamin D. Both these vitamins are "fat-soluble" ones, and they are stored up in the body. And too much is too much. Because vitamin D promotes the absorption of calcium from the intestine, a large stored excess of it can cause excessive quantities of calcium in the blood. What happens then? For one thing, your body's soft tissues may become calcified, or hard. Particularly your kidneys may be the target. And that can mean serious trouble. Eat normally, and you'll avoid this problem.

Vitamin E

Now this is one of the two "super vitamins" health-food fanatics will swear by. And the claims about it go beyond "improving sexual potency."

For instance, in his book *The Heart and Vitamin E and Related Matters*, Dr. Evan Shute (an obstetrician) gives rave reviews to this vitamin and recommends it for the prevention and treatment of an array of unrelated conditions from gangrene and nephritis to varicose veins. But the primary usefulness of vitamin E, according to Dr. Shute and his associates, was in the treatment and prevention of heart disease. Is there any basis to this claim? No, unfortunately there is not. The American Heart Association, the American Medical Association and the Food and Drug Administration, among other groups, have all reported that vitamin E has no value in heart disease or in any other condition with the exception of vitamin E deficiency. So who are you going to believe? One obstetrician or thousands of medical scientists and cardiologists who have professionally evaluated the question and reached a unanimous decision? Or perhaps you favor the many testimonials from those who claim they are now in excellent health after taking vitamin E, but this is not evidence.

According to the National Academy of Sciences, only two types of individuals benefit from supplemental vitamin E therapy: premature babies who may have received inadequate amounts of vitamin E before birth, and persons with intestinal disorders where fats are poorly absorbed. If you're not in either of those categories, forget it—leave the vitamin E capsules off your shopping list.

Can you do any harm by taking this "in" vitamin to keep up with the fad? Possibly. Vitamin E, like A and D, is a fat-soluble vitamin, and a form of toxicity could develop. We know that when it is used in excess, vitamin E has caused headache, nausea, fatigue, giddiness and blurred vision in some people. But not very much is known now about what some long-term, more serious effects overdoses of it might have. So if you insist on being a vitamin E freak, be aware that you are taking part in a massive, uncontrolled experiment.

Vitamin C (Ascorbic Acid)

Vitamin E is only rivaled by vitamin C in the vitamin popularity polls these days.

The real controversy about vitamin C occurred a few years ago when Nobel Prize winner Professor Linus C. Pauling presented his theory that massive doses of vitamin C would both prevent and cure colds. There was a great flurry of interest in his ideas and in his popular book on the subject, and a great deal of professional criticism of his claims. The *Journal of the American Public Health Association* criticized him for making such an announcement in a popular book, as opposed to a professional medical journal, stating:

> Professor Pauling would have been more prudent and would have rendered a greater public service had he presented his ideas to the scientific world for evaluation before recommending them to the public as a basis of action.

As Professor Pauling himself explains in the introduction of his most recent book, *Vitamin C, The Common Cold and the Flu:*

> The idea that I should write a book about vitamin C began to develop in my mind about ten years ago. In April 1966 I received a letter from Irwin Stone, a biochemist whom I had met at the Carl Neuberg Medal Award dinner in New York the previous month. He mentioned in his letter that I had expressed a desire to live for the next 15 or 20 years. He said that he would like to see me remain in good health for the next *fifty* years, and that he was, accordingly, sending me a description of his high-level ascorbic acid regimen, which he had developed during the preceding three decades. My wife and I began the regimen recommended by Stone. We noticed an increased feeling of well-being and especially a striking decrease in the number of colds that we caught, and in their severity.

As a result of this personal success (testimony, not factual evidence) with the vitamin, Professor Pauling pursued the topic of vitamin C and its relationship to disease and made it the focus of the best-selling 1970 book and of this 1976 follow-up version. The central thesis of both works is that large daily doses of vitamin C (250 mg to 5,000 mg) will offer protection from the common cold and that larger doses (5,000 mg to 20,000 mg a day) taken at the first sign that a cold is developing will relieve its symptoms.

To the uncritical reader, the current book will prove quite convincing. It's written in an easy, flowing, appealing style and only rarely becomes tangled in scientific lingo and discussions of statistical association. Pauling has obviously dug deep into the literature on vitamin C and offers his readers some fascinating (albeit, not fully relevant) overviews of the discovery of vitamins, the conquest of scurvy, and the philosophy of "orthomolecular" medicine. The Pauling thesis is well couched in an impressive scientific context of the relationship of nutrition and health.

On the other hand, *Vitamin C, The Common Cold and the Flu* suffers from a problem typical of most polemical presentations, one where the author starts out with a conclusion and proceeds to offer "evidence" to back up his stance. He does not tell his readers the whole story about vitamin C and disease. He tells only the part he wants them to know. For example, after rehashing old and somewhat ambiguous data (a study by Cowen, Diehl and Baker published in 1942, for example), he goes on to say that since the publication of his book in 1970, "several excellent double-blind studies have been carried out." The first of these studies he mentions was conducted in Toronto and, as Pauling notes, the study "involved 407 subjects receiving ascorbic acid (1,000 mg a day plus 3,000 mg a day at the onset of any illness) and 411 subjects receiving a closely matched placebo .... The number of days confined to the house per subject was 30 percent less for the ascorbic acid group than for the placebo group ...." But what Pauling does *not* mention is that the authors of this same study reported *no* statistically significant differences between the two groups in the total number of episodes of illness and, similarly, no difference in the total number of days of recorded symptoms. In other parts of his book he mentions, but then dismisses, the results of controlled studies which do not support his argument on the basis of "methodological problems," in this case, an allegedly inadequate placebo.

Of even more concern is the incomplete story-telling in Pauling's chapter entitled "The Side Effects of Vitamin C." Indeed, in this section he makes a rather extraordinary statement: "Ascorbic acid ... is safe, even when taken in very large amounts, far larger than the amounts that are needed to combat the common cold." Judging from his earlier pronouncements, then, Pauling has declared daily doses of 20,000 milligrams or more unequivocably "safe." Given that data on the medical sequelae of long-term overdosing of vitamin C are just now being accumulated, this conclusion appears unjustified. Indeed, given that the scientific method calls for testing for harmful effects as opposed to establishing absolute safety, such a statement is probably never appropriate.

Pauling quickly passes off reports that large doses of vitamin C taken with food can destroy the vitamin B_{12} in food, leading to a deficiency disease resembling pernicious anemia. While he briefly discusses and, again, dismisses the possible rebound effect with vitamin C, he does not mention the potential problems of vitamin C overdosing during pregnancy and the possibility that the newborn child will suffer from scurvy despite normal intake of vitamin C. Instead his chapter on side effects communicates the general message: "All the warnings about high doses of vitamin C are made by alarmists."

The chapter on vitamin C and its alleged protective effect against influenza is extremely weak. Pauling opens it by acknowledging that there is no epidemiological evidence relating ascorbic acid to decreased illness from influenza, but then goes on to say, "There is, however, little reason to expect it to be less effective than it is with the common cold and other viral diseases." He makes no serious attempt to present any clinical evidence there, and one wonders if mention of the word "flu" in the title of the book, and an inclusion of an eight-page chapter on the subject, were not a promotional ploy taking advantage of the obvious public interest in the subject in January 1977 when the book came on the market.

Probably the most fascinating aspect of this book is not the discussion of vitamin C and disease, but the innuendo throughout that we have here a case of Linus Pauling versus medical and nutritional professionals. He frequently complains that his pronouncements on vitamin C are "ignored," that medical journals refuse to publish his material and that the medical community and federal regulatory agencies reject his hypothesis because they are economically, or in some other personal way, threatened by it. In a chapter entitled "The Medical Establishment and Vitamin C" he writes, "Despite the repeated findings that an increased intake of vitamin C provides some protection against respiratory illness and other diseases . . . our Federal health agencies continue to deny that it has any value."

Of course, the crucial question in any discussion of the new (or previous) Pauling book is "Do high dosages of vitamin C prevent the common cold—or offer some relief from it?"

One can spend hours citing studies and arguing about whether or not they are double-blind, and in other ways adequate, but it seems— at least to us—that the unmistakable "drift" of the many investigations in this area is that there is no evidence that low, medium or high doses of the vitamin will offer protection from respiratory illness, and that while high doses of ascorbic acid may relieve some of the unpleasant symptoms of a cold—particularly feelings of stuffiness and lethargy, a number of different and widely available antihistamines accomplish this end much more efficiently. But despite this, hundreds of thousands of consumers have either read the Pauling book or—more likely—seen and heard him discuss his ideas on television or radio shows and assumed a "well-maybe-he's-right-and-maybe-he's-wrong-but-just-in-case-I-better-buy-some-vitamin-C-capsules" attitude.

It is ironic in this age of chemical phobia that the same consumer who shivers after learning that a product contains a trace of BHA, red dye #40 or nitrite will eagerly gobble extraordinary amounts of a chemical called ascorbic acid.

Is there anything seriously wrong about the ongoing Pauling vs. "established medicine" debate? No—and yes.

"No" in the sense that most consumers will probably follow the traditional drug compliance—or rather, noncompliance—pattern and take their vitamin C tablets only occasionally, not ingesting enough to cause themselves physical harm.

But "yes" in that the controversy is causing a type of unconstructive polarization on the topic of vitamin C and its relationship to health. It *is* possible that ascorbic acid doses above the current RDA may, in some instances, promote health. The full gamut of potential benefits from this vitamin probably has not been identified. Only recently has ascorbic acid received attention in the meat curing process, its capacity for inhibiting nitrosamine formation now being recognized. Perhaps vitamin C *will* play an important role in disease prevention and treatment in the future. One should not categorize himself as a "pro" or "anti" vitamin C advocate. Open-mindedness is the essential ingredient in scientific process, and advances will not occur if all new and unusual ideas are scoffed at. There may be a new horizon for this substance. But right now, after studying the Pauling case for ascorbic acid and relying on the best available methodological binoculars, the prevention for the common cold does not appear to be part of that new horizon.

So the next time you hear Professor Pauling's advice on vitamin C and the common cold, remember that his conclusions do not have the support of the great majority of medical scientists and keep in mind that while Professor Pauling is one of very few people ever to receive the Nobel Prize on two separate occasions (Chemistry and Peace), he is not a physician and not a nutritionist.

Be Healthier and Richer Too! Don't Supplement!

Unless, of course, you have a medical reason to do so. In addition to the possibility of hurting yourself with an overdose, you may inadvertently disguise a sympton which, under normal conditions, would have prompted you to see a physician. Consider a case involving folic acid, one of the important B vitamins.

Investigation into the proper use of this vitamin formed one of the great medical advances of recent years. Countless hours of painstaking research finally revealed that folic acid will relieve many of the symptoms of a disease known as pernicious anemia. It was also learned that this vitamin is useful in the treatment of the anemia of sprue and of certain other conditions in which there is poor absorption of food.

However—and here is the catch—caution has been urged against the use of large amounts of folic acid in vitamin preparations intended for the public. Why? The explanation is fascinating. Although folic acid corrects certain of the symptoms associated with pernicious anemia of man, *it does not stop the progression of disturbances of the nervous system.* Therefore, irreparable damage to the nervous system may occur if an individual, lulled into thinking he has been cured because the anemia has responded to the folic acid, fails to seek medical attention. When the error is finally discovered, it may be too late for the damage to the nervous system to be properly treated.

It is clear, then, that if a vitamin is needed as medication it should be obtained through a physician. On the whole, however, today vitamins are needed, not to cure disease, but to build health, and plenty are obtained from a well-balanced varied diet.

What About Iron?

Do women need more iron than men?

The answer is yes; because of periodic blood loss and the added demands of childbearing, women do need more iron than men. Reliable estimates show that in the United States three out of every five women have some degree of iron deficiency.

What does this mean? Do most women need to resort to pills and medication?

Luckily the answer is no, because the normal iron requirement can be met by a well-balanced diet. Unluckily, though, women tend to skimp on this important mineral, for they often have just juice and coffee for breakfast, "anything that happens to be around" for lunch, and the small end of the family's meat dish in the evening.

Iron-rich foods can, however, be included in every meal, and they are essential not only for women but for everyone. Rich, red, healthy blood needs iron. When the iron supply is low the blood cannot do its job of carrying oxygen to the body cells. Also, iron is necessary for the production of certain enzymes that help change food into body energy. As we mentioned in chapter two, one of the best sources of iron is liver. This contains not only iron but many other highly nutritious constituents. Liver in the menu even as seldom as twice a month benefits the whole family. All kinds of liver are good—beef and calf, pork, chicken and lamb—and it can be served in many ways: baked, broiled, chopped, or ground and combined with beef as loaf or meatballs. Eat iron from liver and the other sources mentioned earlier, and you probably won't need pills! But if you are definitely anemic, your physician will treat the anemia with an iron preparation, and when the hemoglobin is back to where it should be, you can keep it there with a proper diet.

THERE'S MORE GOODNESS THAN EVER BEFORE IN OUR FOODS

But you'd never believe it if you accepted everything you read in newspapers these days, or hear on radio and TV. The poisons you hear so much about are actually in the pens of a small group of individuals in this country who have committed themselves to the cause of convincing American eaters that we are the victims of over-processed, "empty" junk foods produced by greedy, uncaring food manufacturers. In part the motivation is ego building, for they get publicity, and in part economic because such ideas when put into books sell well.

The height of the nonsense was an annual event called "Food Day," first launched in the spring of 1975. Organized by a microbiologist who is co-director of the "Center for Science in the Public Interest," Food Day was planned to crack down on what the planners called "the terrible ten," foods chosen allegedly because they "exemplify what's wrong with American food." Interestingly, one of their condemned foods was the good old-fashioned natural table grape. Why? Because of union problems between the United Farm Workers and grape pickers in California. Now that's not exactly what we call nutritionally sound reasoning!

And the other nine sentenced-to-oblivion foods?: bacon, allegedly because it contains a "dangerous additive," nitrite (despite the fact that nitrite added to foods has never been shown to pose a health hazard to man and, indeed, is present in a number of very "natural" substances such as spinach, other leafy green vegetables, radishes, celery—and human saliva); prime-grade beef because "it is high in fat, price and cholesterol content" (In condemning this plentiful and delicious source of protein, the Food Day planners were clearly irresponsible and uninformed, as many substances in our diet contain significant amounts of cholesterol, some appreciably more than beef, but all contribute to good health when used in moderation); Wonder Bread (because it is baked by a division of ITT and ITT also makes military supplies—again, another piece of "nutritional genius"); and Coca-Cola, Breakfast Squares, Gerber Baby Food Desserts, Fruit Brute (a dry cereal), Pringles (a potato chip) and good old-fashioned sugar, all got the "unapproved" rating even though all these products are unquestionably safe for human consumption, contribute significantly to eating enjoyment and fit in with our fast-paced lifestyle. Certainly none of the foods on the "Terrible Ten" or any other list of foods should be used to excess—or allowed to replace the foods in the essential Basic Four. But to condemn all of them? Ridiculous and, again, very irresponsible.

Subsequent Food Days condemned individuals and organizations which allegedly contributed to poor nutrition in the U.S. (the senior author of this book made the list!) and expanded an earlier criticism of so-called "empty calories" and "junk food."

You'll keep hearing diatribes about how "unfit" the American food supply is. What is tragic is not that there are people who make these statements. There have *always* been fringe individuals who, under the guise of "consumer interests," make their career out of attacking the food supply—or any other vulnerable subject, for that matter. But what is both puzzling and disappointing is the fact that the press and other news media, and various members of Congress, give so much attention to these unscientific statements. Perhaps if consumers informed their local media representatives that they were interested in food facts, nutritional sense and not nonsense, we'd all be better off.

Let's look at some of the common charges made against our food supply which, beyond doubt is one of the best, if not the best, in the world.

Brown vs. White Sugar vs. No Sugar

"It's best not to eat sugar at all, but if you have to, stick to 'natural' sugar!" That's a basic premise of the proponents of health-food-land. Does it make any sense? No—but then most everything else they say about nutritional differences between "regular" and "health food" is off-base too.

Raw or unrefined sugar has been a food of continuing faddist focus. Just what the nutritional merits of brown sugar are is somewhat vague, it being generally described as "good for maintaining vigor." But then there is the possibility that some snob appeal may be operative too, because brown sugar is significantly more expensive than the white refined type in common use.

Analyses of brown sugar versus white sugar reveal that there is, indeed, slightly more nutritive value in the brown type. One tablespoon of brown sugar contains 1/24th as much calcium as one glass of milk, or to extend this useful bit of information, an adult needs only three cups of brown sugar a day to provide his body with sufficient calcium. There is no need to point out to those with a weight problem that these three cups of brown sugar provide 2,400 Calories, more than enough to cause a weight gain in a sedentary adult. That's before the brown-sugar craver even starts out to meet his daily Basic Four!

Aside from the calcium in brown sugar, there is also some iron. By computation, adult women can meet their daily requirement of iron by eating only two and one-half cups of brown sugar.

These figures clearly show that brown sugar, despite the presence of a speck more calcium and iron than is found in white sugar, is not of nutritional importance except (as all sugars) as a source of carbohydrates. And what about vitamins in brown sugar? Vitamins A and C are totally absent and so little of the B vitamins is present that we must refer to it as a "trace." So forget the brown sugar for daily use, unless you prefer its taste. And, of course, use it when your special dessert recipes call for it!

But what about sugar generally? Should you classify it as a junk food and throw out all your sugar bowls?

No! We'll discuss sugar in more detail when we turn our attention to the so-called "McGovern Report" on U.S. dietary goals. But here we'll simply state that sugar is an efficient, low-cost source of calories which, you recall, we need for energy. Besides, it makes many foods taste good. And remember that eating is supposed to be fun! You've heard rumors about sugar causing diabetes and heart disease? Not so! Even in excess amounts, sugar is not a cause of diabetes. Obesity is the big nutritional hazard of the diabetic, regardless of the source of the calories.

A number of scientific reviews on the subject of sugar and heart disease have come up with negative findings. There is no good evidence today that these two are linked. We've already issued a pardon to sugar consumed with meals in the case of dental decay, but it's worth repeating here for emphasis: for some people sugar may accelerate dental decay, but it is the sticky excessive sugar consumption taken between meals which is involved in the acceleration of decay, not the sugar with meals. And there is only one practical way today to deal with the problem of tooth decay and that is fluoridated water early in life and till death do us part.

White vs. Brown Bread

For centuries a topic of conversation for the average eater, and particularly of the food faddist, has been whether the "staff of life" should be white or brown. An overwhelming majority of voters have cast their votes for white bread. Even the Greeks had a word for it.

The dark-bread aficionados extoll the merits of whole wheat and predict dire fates for the users of white-flour products. Yet most people continue to eat white bread. And their reason? Simply because they like it.

The controversy between white and brown bread began in earnest in the United States about a century ago with a Massachusetts clergyman named Sylvester Graham. The impression created by Reverend Graham's endorsement of "unbolted wheat-meal flour" was so great that the products he eulogized, Graham flour, Graham crackers, and Graham bread still bear his name.

Whole-meal bread was good, he said, because it was "natural" and "vital." He condemned the practice of separating the flour from the bran as "to put asunder that which God has joined together."

White flour must have been rather commonly used at the time Graham lived, otherwise there would have been no need for his so-called "branny" campaign.

People's taste preferences for bread have not changed appreciably through the centuries. Despite the dire predictions of faddists and in spite of extensive and expensive advertising campaigns to sell whole-wheat flour, white bread continues to outsell whole-grain bread by five to one.

You'll still hear that white bread is "fattening, overprocessed, worthless, full of air and additives." It is true that some vitamins and minerals are lost when the bran and wheat germ are removed from the flour. What faddists fail to point out, however, is that most flour today is fortified with thiamine, riboflavin, niacin and iron. As you can see from the table below, enriched white bread and whole-wheat are essentially nutritionally identical:

	White Enriched (1 average slice)	Whole-Wheat (1 average slice)
Calories	63	55
Protein, grams	2.0	2.1
Carbohydrates, grams	11.9	11.3
Fat, grams	.7	.6
Iron, milligrams	.4	.5
Thiamine, milligrams	.06	.07
Riboflavin, milligrams	.04	.03
Niacin, milligrams	.5	.7

The plea for the use of whole-wheat flour and bread in the average American diet today does not have nutritional justification, but it is a good way of increasing the fiber content of the diet.

Americans are blessed with an abundance of nutritious foods. In such a varied and healthful diet, whole-wheat flour and its products have not been proved to be superior to enriched refined (white) flour.

On the other hand, whole-wheat bread is nutritious and good. So if you like dark bread, eat and enjoy it. Bread, white or dark, is important in our diets, is part of the Basic Four, and is as "good" nutritionally as it ever was. And any store that sells bread or other foods is a health-food store!

Fresh vs. Frozen vs. Canned

Which has a higher vitamin content? Home canned, commercially canned, frozen or fresh vegetables, fruits and juices?

For all practical purposes in our varied diets they are essentially the same. Fresh produce, if really fresh, like the corn, tomatoes or strawberries you may pick in your own garden, have a maximum nutrient value (they also taste really good!), that is, if you pick them at just the right time and cook them properly—which you cannot always do. These latter reasons are why commercially processed foods are frequently superior in nutritive value: they are harvested and processed scientifically. But, in practice, as part of our total dietary pattern, all are equally nutritious. Tastes and appearance may vary widely, but not nutritive values.

But what about fruit juices? Do they vary in nutrient content if they are frozen, bottled, canned or freshly squeezed?

Again, a comparison of average nutrient content for frozen, canned and fresh orange juice shows that there is little difference between the three methods of preparation. For example, the following figures compare the amount of the vitamin C in 100 grams (3½ ounces) of orange juice prepared by the three methods. The primary nutritional purpose of including citrus in our diet is to meet our vitamin C requirements.

Orange Juice Type	Vitamin C Content
Fresh	50 milligrams
Canned	40 milligrams
Frozen	45 milligrams

Again, for all practical purposes, these are equal. But no one is denying that when you have access to oranges, freshly squeezed juice is mighty good!

Just an additional note about orange juice. Be sure to distinguish between synthetic frozen concentrates and various orangeades and pops. The latter items are not intended to simulate full strength of orange juice. But the synthetic juices do. It seems that the chemists figured out a way to make vitamin C cheaper than nature's very own oranges and grapefruit can. If vitamin C is added to an orangeade or a noncitrus fruit juice at a level comparable to those in the table above, it is equally nutritious to orange juice when used in a diet of varied foods based around the Basic Four Food Groups. Read the label!

Is Processing Preferable?

In many cases—in view of our desire for quick foods, and foods with long shelf lives—yes!

But the term "processed" has raised concerns. Health-food promoters describe this category of foods as "natural foods which have been adulterated in some way to deceive the consumer and make extra money for the manufacturer." But before you panic, consider what the term "processing" really is. In its broadest sense, any product which is treated in any way after it leaves the farm is processed. Pasteurizing milk makes it a processed product. And in speaking of processing, why doesn't anyone ever mention the benefits and convenience processed products offer to the consumer?

"What about instant mashed potatoes," some people ask, "are they as nutritious as mashed potatoes made from scratch?" And the answer is simple:

Potatoes are good food and instant mashed potatoes are one of the great convenient foods of these times. Nutritionally speaking, potatoes are largely carbohydrate (starch), but they do contain small amounts of protein and are a fairly good source of vitamin C. The latter is well-retained in potatoes boiled in their jackets but is lost when the potatoes are beaten up with air as in mashed potatoes. As far as the carbohydrate and protein content, it would be essentially the same in either instant mashed or "old-fashioned" mashed potatoes. Many of the instant mashed potatoes have vitamin C added. Again, read the label.

But what about the difference between instant oatmeal and regular oatmeal?

Again, there is no difference from a nutritional value: both are identical and both are good for you. Regular rolled oats are prepared by steaming the entire oat groat and passing it between steel rolls to produce a flake. To produce the quick cooking or instant form, the oat groat is first cut into several pieces and those individual pieces then steamed and rolled out. This produces a thinner flake. In turn, more of the starch is exposed, and the cooking process is quicker simply because it is mechanically easier for the hot water to reach the starch granules.

One of the much maligned processed foods is processed cheese. Definitely on the forbidden list for the committed food faddist. But what is cheese processing?

It's actually not much more complicated than pasteurizing—processing—milk. The manufacturer mixes together a number of different hard cheeses (to ensure uniformity and flavor from batch to batch), heats them to a point of pasteurization and pours them into molds to cool. Because natural cheese separates into its component parts when it is heated, an emulsifier, usually a type of phosphate, is added to the mixture in a homogenized state. Phosphates! Additives! But wait! Phosphorus is an essential element of all human life, animal and vegetable, and despite what your local food faddist says to the contrary, there is no reason to believe that it is anything but a health-promoting substance. Heating the cheese, adding phosphates so it stays mixed (not more than 3 percent phosphates are allowed by law) and cooling it in the desired shape—that's all cheese processing is about. Occasionally some salt is added if the natural cheese is lacking it, and possibly up to 1 percent water is used for consistency. But the whole process is as natural as you can get. You probably are already familiar with a major advantage of processed cheese—unlike hard cheese it keeps almost indefinitely in your refrigerator, maintaining its uniform taste and texture. And since it has been pasteurized, it doesn't even need to be always refrigerated.

The new nutritional labels are proving to be a great help to us in understanding the nutritive value in different types of processed food. For instance, in buying rice, you'll want to study the label closely, taking into account the relative importance to you of three factors: cost, nutritive value and cooking time. Brown rice is a good source of B vitamins and a few other nutrients; but it can take some time to prepare, and some people don't like it as much as fluffy white rice. So-called "minute rices" are more expensive, quick-cooking and of somewhat lower nutritive value. "Parboiled rice" is much better nutritionally and compares favorably with the nutrition of brown rice. Its advantages are that it cooks in about half the time required to soften the bran layer of the brown rice, but on the other hand, it is not as quickly prepared as the "quick" rices, and it is relatively expensive.

In some cities you can buy an enriched polished rice which is made by mixing two types of polished rice, one of which has been coated with a vitamin premix containing thiamine, riboflavin, niacin and iron. If you can find this type, buy it!

And when you cook either parboiled, enriched or brown rice, since they are good sources of the water soluble vitamin B (thiamine), it is important to prepare them in just enough water so that there is only a trace of moistness in the bottom of the pan.

Milk: Whole, Skim, Evaporated, "99% Fat Free" and Chocolate

Milk is an excellent source of calcium, riboflavin, protein, phosphorus and thiamine. But you can drink it in a number of forms.

Skim milk, as its name suggests, has had its fat removed. That by definition means that its fat-soluble vitamin A has also been removed. But the majority of today's skim milk has been fortified with vitamin A (read the label) so that's no problem. Skim milk is a marvelous food for the diet—rich in nutrients without all the calories of regular milk.

You've undoubtedly seen the milks which are labeled "99% fat free" on your supermarket dairy shelf. These milks have become very popular in recent years in that they are a compromise between whole milk and skim milk. Some of the fat is left behind so the product has more the texture of "regular" milk. But the question is, how much fat is left? The answer, as the name of the product implies, is that 1 percent is left. But don't be fooled. Regular whole milk is 97 percent fat free. So don't be overwhelmed by the advertising. What you are buying here is a quart with 1 to 2 percent fat, as opposed to the usual 3 to 3½ percent fat. A more reasonable way to promote these milks would be to say that 66 percent of the fat has been removed! But Madison Avenue doesn't see it that way. Compare the calorie counts of milk and choose on the basis of your needs.

Calories Per Cup

Whole milk	160
Nonfat (skim)	90
Partly skimmed (99% fat free)	145

Many of the 1 percent milks (99 percent fat free) have 2 percent skimmed milk solids added. This not only improves the taste and "body" of the milk but also improves it nutritionally, because the skim milk solids include the protein, minerals, and water soluble vitamins of the milk.

Evaporated milk is canned milk which has approximately half its water removed. When it is opened and mixed with an equal amount of water, it is comparable to fresh milk. It can be used successfully in puddings and other desserts, creamed soups, creamed sauces, scrambled eggs and baked goods. But remember to use half as much milk as the recipe calls for and add an equal amount of water. In contrast to evaporated milk, sweetened condensed milk is made by evaporating just about half the water from whole milk and adding a great deal of sugar to keep it from spoiling. After a while on your shelves, you may notice that sweetened condensed milk begins to look like caramel, but it is still good food—if you like the taste.

Canned and dried milks are good to keep around because of their long shelf life. Your family doesn't like powdered milk? Use it in your cooking when the recipe calls for a cup of milk—and mix it in with regular milk. They won't know the difference, the nutritional quality will be the same, and you'll be saving money too.

And no discussion of milk is complete without mentioning that all-time childhood favorite, chocolate milk. Is it just as acceptable to substitute chocolate milk for white milk?

Actually arguments can be made for both sides of the case. First, however, it would seem necessary to define the products we are talking about. Chocolate milk and chocolate dairy drink are a little different in composition, and we hasten to add that the latter is the one most frequently available on the commercial market.

Chocolate milk must be made from whole milk with a butterfat content of not less than 3.25 percent, while the dairy drink is made from skim or partially skimmed milk and has a butterfat content of about 2.0 percent. For this reason, the dairy drink is a less expensive product. A further difference is in the caloric content. Chocolate dairy drink has more calories than an equal amount of whole milk, and chocolate milk has even a few more calories.

Both have chocolate syrup or powder, some sugar and stabilizers added. As you probably noticed, they tend to have a rather thick and viscous consistency. This is due to the addition of the stabilizers, such as carageenin, a seaweed extract. Many health claims have been made for chocolate flavored milk, but there have also been protests that adding chocolate to milk may render some of the nutrients unavailable for human absorption. The latter is not true, and it is safe to say that chocolate milk or dairy drink contribute the nutrients available in the milk from which it was made.

Then, what are some of the practical considerations governing the allowance of chocolate milk? First, one might consider the child's weight. It is obviously poor practice to encourage the overweight child to drink chocolate milk with more calories when skim milk, whole milk or a mixture of part skim and part whole milk would provide the nutrients he needs, with fewer calories. Second, one would want to discourage the use of chocolate milk or chocolate dairy drink in children who have poor appetites. Sugar and sweets, particularly when taken shortly before a meal, tend to depress the appetite, and a child who doesn't care too much about food may frequently drink his chocolate milk and forego lunch! Finally, chocolate is occasionally implicated as a culprit in childhood allergies and in some cases of adolescent acne. Should this be the case, one would, of course, not want to give chocolate to such a child.

For the average child of normal weight, who has a good appetite and no apparent sensitivity to chocolate, there is no harm in allowing chocolate milk or chocolate dairy drink for part of his daily milk consumption. And certainly, since milk is an important food in a child's diet, those few who insist on chocolate should be permitted to have it. Better chocolate milk than no milk at all!

While we're speaking about milk, a brief comment on a very popular milk product might be in order.

The nutritional value of ice creams is directly related to the amount of milk, cream and sugar they contain. Ice cream has what is called a "standard of identity," that is, to call a product ice cream it must have a definite level of milk fat and of certain other ingredients. The somewhat similar products developed in recent years cannot be called ice creams because they do not meet these standards. Generally these products have less fat and milk and are called "freezes," custards, or frozen puddings. They have less nutritive value because of less fat and milk. Also, they usually contain more air which of course dilutes the nutritive value. Price might be a good clue in choosing among various products. If a half gallon of a product calls for about the same price as a pint of another, it means it has far less milk and fat, and more air, per serving, than the more expensive ice cream. But if you are trying to cut down on calories this type of dessert would be preferred.

Enriched? Fortified? Imitation?

Chances are that if you went into the kitchen right now, you'd find these words liberally sprinkled all over your food. But what do they mean? Enrichment means that nutrients such as thiamine, riboflavin, iron, and niacin have been added to make up for some of those nutrients removed by processing.

Fortification is a more general term which refers to the addition of specific vitamins and minerals to food, often where they were not in the first place. For instance, our common table salt is generally fortified with iodide. Milks are fortified with vitamin D, margarines with vitamins A and D, and some breads with calcium and vitamin D.

You are probably noticing more and more foods labeled "food substitute" or "imitation" on your supermarket shelves. For instance you can now find an "imitation" mayonnaise and imitation margarine which have the advantage of offering a taste comparable to the regular products—but half the calories. Additionally, the high cost of meat has caused consumers all over the country to look into various blends of ground beef and textured vegetable protein which resembles the nutritive value of beef but is lower in cost due to the substitution of plant protein for some of the animal beef protein. Each supermarket has its own variety and way of packaging the burger mix. Some sell a packet containing soy and wheat protein concentrates and a variety of herbs and spices. The packet is added to regular ground beef and is then used in cooking as one would use ground beef. Another market may sell the beef premixed.

Either type of product is a bargain for the consumer. In addition, the beef-soy blends are lower in fat content than pure beef. With our present knowledge of the relationship of high animal fat diets to coronary heart disease, eating these newer combination beef-vegetable protein mixtures may, in the long run, be more beneficial to our health than always eating pure animal meat.

How do you use these burger mixtures? A hamburger made from the mix tastes very much like a burger made from pure ground beef, though the texture may not be quite the same. The burger mixtures work particularly well in mixed dishes such as casseroles and meatballs or loafs where the juiciness characteristic of a hamburger is not anticipated.

PLAY IT SAFE—PROTECT YOUR FOOD!

Look around your grocery or drug store and note the hundreds of items stocked there. Have you ever stopped to consider what is involved in protecting the purity of all these products?

Anyone who remembers the fly-covered foods of earlier decades, anyone who has seen the lack of sanitation in many other countries, can appreciate the carefully packaged and displayed products we now enjoy in the United States. This is no simple accomplishment! In fact, it requires a vast network of highly-trained people working in many specialized agencies.

These activities were reviewed not long ago by the Committee on Nutrition of the American Academy of Pediatrics. To read about them is reassuring for every consumer. Even a brief summary helps one realize how much is being done to guarantee the quality and safety of our nation's food.

The *Food and Drug Administration* is responsible for establishing and maintaining many important standards. Some of its areas include: (1) food purity and honest labeling, (2) regulation of use of additives and pesticides, (3) inspection of plants and food and drug shipments, and (4) monitoring of toxicity and radioactivity of foods. In addition, the Food and Drug Administration has a Bureau of Scientific Research, to foster further work in this whole important area.

The *United States Public Health Service* is another guarantor of the safety of our food. Its federal, state, and local offices supervise such aspects of public health as (1) ordinances and codes for the handling of milk and other products, (2) air and water pollution, (3) contamination of foods and other sanitation problems, and (4) prevention of radiological hazards. The Public Health Service also supports pertinent research in many universities and hospitals.

The *United States Department of Agriculture* watches over billions of pounds of meat and poultry. Thus consumers may be sure of a product which is clean and without disease, and which is free of hazards from radioactivity, from pesticides, and from drug residues.

The *Atomic Energy Commission* also supervises levels of radioactive substances. The chairman of this commission, along with the secretaries of Defense, Labor, Commerce, and of Health, Education and Welfare have established "Radiation Protection Guides" so that foods can be safeguarded from radioactive contamination.

Nongovernmental groups also give valuable assistance. The National Research Council maintains a Food and Nutrition Board which deals with many aspects of public health nutrition, including food protection. Both the American Academy of Pediatrics and the American Medical Association have Nutrition Committees that are concerned with food standards. In addition, many of the larger food, chemical, and drug companies, as well as many other manufacturers, are constantly developing tests and processes to improve food production and safety.

But When You Get Home, It's Up to You!

Food is a dynamic entity. It changes over time, and some of those changes can threaten your health, if only to give you a bellyache.

Food spoils in a number of ways. In what is known as microbial food spoilage, bacteria, yeasts or molds develop. You've seen the fuzzy growth on spoiled bread, cheese and on the surface of jams and jellies that you've had around too long. You're also familiar with the type of microbial food spoilage characteristic of sour milk or spoiled eggs.

Another type of spoilage is an enzymic type, which results in more of a loss of quality of the food as opposed to making them inedible. Frozen vegetables you keep around for many months may acquire a haylike flavor which is hardly enhancing to an enjoyable meal.

Third, there is chemical spoilage, better known as oxidation, the kind of changes you notice when you peel a potato or apple and leave it in its raw state without benefit of water.

How do you avoid food spoilage? Obviously part of the answer is to not let your food supply sit around too long after you purchase it. Another way is to take proper freezing and refrigeration precautions to maximize the shelf-life of your various foods. Take your groceries right home. Don't let them sit in the car in the hot sun while you do your errands, and make sure your refrigerator is between thirty-five to forty degrees.

So part of food safety is the prevention of or delay of spoilage and adherence to the age-old rule, "When in doubt, throw it out." If your nose detects some unusual smell, or if a food begins to look "funny," why risk your family's health to find out if it's safe or not?

Another basic of food safety is cooking food that needs to be cooked. We'll discuss the pork question next, but here it is important to note that you shouldn't let any meat sit in the oven for several hours before the oven is programmed to begin heating the food. Most meats that are strictly fresh can be left two hours in a cold oven, and frozen meats will survive longer, but it is generally unwise, for instance, to put a roast in the oven as you leave for work, have the oven go on automatically in the afternoon, and plan to arrive home for a health-promoting dinner.

And speaking of meats, for your health's sake, don't experiment by eating raw meat. For instance, raw ground sirloin, with or without the fat, can cause worms if the meat is contaminated with the beef tapeworm. This is the most common tapeworm found in man in the United States. It can be harmful, and it should be treated. Cook your meat to be on the safe side. And if you have some left over from dinner, refrigerate it. Don't let it stand at room temperature for prolonged periods of time.

Watch Out for the Two S's

Salmonella and staphylococci. They both spell trouble if they multiply in your food.

Salmonella is the scientific name of a large group of microscopic organisms (bacteria) found almost everywhere that man or animals exist. To date, over 1200 strains of this bacteria have been isolated, all of which can cause infection in man and animals.

But what is salmonellosis? How does one get it? What are some preventive measures against it? We can begin explaining that the disease is caused by the salmonella bacteria, which enter the body in the food we eat or in the milk and water we drink. These organisms have been found in a variety of foods and beverages, ranging from dried milk and eggs to watermelons that have been grown in contaminated soil!

These bacteria cause trouble because they liberate a toxin which irritates the lining of the digestive tract, cause a low fever, nausea, vomiting, diarrhea and abdominal cramps. Although the acute symptoms disappear rather rapidly, the infected individual may become a "carrier" of these bacteria and be a source of infection for others. Such a person, employed as a food handler, represents a serious potential problem. For this reason, employees who handle food should have regular medical checkups. But infected food handlers, however, are only one of the possible modes of salmonella infection.

Frequently for instance, the organisms are found in raw or unprocessed foods. Chickens, which have been given contaminated feed, may harbor the bacteria in their flesh. Fish caught in polluted waters are another frequent source of infection. And, one of the biggest problems is the egg. Fresh, frozen and dried eggs have all been known to carry salmonella organisms. In fact, the federal goverment has set up stringent requirements for processing eggs to minimize infection from this source.

Rats, rodents and insects such as the common housefly may carry salmonella organisms and contaminate clean food. Even improperly cleaned food-handling equipment can transmit salmonella. For example, a slicing machine in a neighborhood delicatessen was found to be the source of a large outbreak of salmonella infection.

This all sounds rather dismal, but much can be done about it. Food manufacturers have a vital interest in reducing the risk of salmonella infection. They are constantly studying ways to build safeguards into their production systems. Manufacturers of commercial equipment must cooperate to design machinery that can be easily and thoroughly cleaned. Many businesses and institutions which employ food handlers have regular health-screening programs to eliminate salmonella carriers, and all should have.

The federal government continues to be actively involved in fighting the problem. They are engaged in research and investigation to set sensible requirements for manufacturers to follow in order to reduce the risk of salmonella infection.

And finally, you can do your share to protect your own family. Here are some simple rules to follow:

1. Refrigerate all perishable foods. This is especially important when you're preparing a roast turkey. Don't let it sit around thawed while you make the dressing. And incidentally, don't stuff your bird until you're ready to put it in a preheated oven.
2. Refrigerate cooked foods promptly! Prolonged cooling at room temperature provides an excellent medium for bacterial growth. Again, take special care with turkey and other fowl.
3. Cover all foods on open counters. Keep stored foods in containers that are inaccessible to any stray mouse that wanders in out of the blue!
4. Cook food thoroughly. When possible, heat prepared foods.
5. "When in doubt, throw it out!"

The adjective "ubiquitous" has often been used to describe salmonella. This is just a fancy way of saying, "They're everywhere." However, through joint efforts by industry, government, and the consumer, the threat of salmonella infection can be reduced to a minimum.

The staphylococcus bacteria are responsible for many cases of food poisoning each year. The toxin involved affects only the gastrointestinal tract and the onset of the symptoms occur within two to twelve hours after the infected food is eaten. The symptoms include severe nausea, vomiting and abdominal cramps. Succinctly stated, it makes the victim pretty miserable for a few hours. Too often the misery sets in after a fun-filled summer afternoon picnic.

So remember, hot weather plus picnics may equal trouble—but it needn't! The trouble is, most picnic foods are as well liked by germs as by people, and picnic weather is as fine for germs as for people.

The way to avoid trouble? Follow a few common sense rules.

1. If you have any doubts about a food, don't use it!
2. Cold foods must be thoroughly chilled and kept that way.
3. Hot foods must be piping hot and kept that way.
4. Never let cooked foods cool down to room temperature on the kitchen counter or on the picnic table. Refrigerate while still hot.
5. Use sanitized utensils for mixing foods—*never* your hands— and sanitized containers for transporting foods.
6. Invest in a good insulated cooler if you must picnic farther away than your own backyard.

The germs that cause most stomach upsets are found everywhere— on our skin, in the diet, in the air. They are easily destroyed by cooking temperatures and are inactivated by cold. They thrive from about 50° to 140° Fahrenheit. Once they have been allowed to grow in food and produce their toxin, cooking or chillling won't help much.

What are safe picnic foods? Raw fruits and vegetables that have been thoroughly washed and kept cool; baked beans, potato chips, most beverages except milk; anything in a tin or jar that has not been opened, such as salmon, tuna, sardines, pickles, relishes, potato salad, macaroni salad, spaghetti and meatballs, fruits, and juices; meat for grilling, such as hamburgers, franks, steak, chicken, ham, that has been thoroughly chilled or even frozen at home and transported in a cold chiller; cooked meats such as chicken, ham, luncheon meat, and meat loaf that have been well chilled at home and carried in a chiller. A good plan is to have all cooked meats in the cooking pan—it has been sterilized by the cooking heat. Chill the cooking pan and carry the meat in the pan, carefully wrapped.

Unsafe foods? Better avoid that special potato salad or those elegant deviled eggs unless you have used very careful procedures in making them, and unless they can be kept cold. Of course, never, never take cream or custard pies, cream puffs, eclairs, whipped-cream cake, Boston cream pie, and cheesecake. These foods are asking for trouble. Save them for home eating!

Being Safe Instead of Sorry

Any discussion of food safety must at least touch on two dreaded types of food contamination, trichinosis and botulism. Given our country's high standards of food safety the overwhelming odds are that you'll never have to have a real concern about these problems, but there are some basic facts you ought to know.

Occasionally pigs are fed untreated garbage and, as a result, the animals harbor a parasite known as *Trichinella spiralis*. Generally however, the feed is treated in a way to make the presence of this parasite impossible. But there remains the slim possibility it may turn up in the pork chop or pork shoulders you buy. To avoid any possibility of illness, cook your pork products thoroughly! Be sure, at the very least, that you make sure all the "pink" is gone from the meat. Don't worry about certain pork products like bacon and sausage which are designed to cook in a very short time. These have been treated in a fashion which ensures that the offending parasites, if present at all, are dead.

Then there is botulism, a disease you usually only hear about in the public media—and then only rarely—when food manufacturers are recalling canned products which *might* be contaminated. Fortunately these are rare occurrences today.

The disease agent *Clostridium botulinum* can only grow in the absence of air. And as it grows it produces a powerful deadly toxin, more deadly than venom from a cobra. As little as 0.01 milligrams of this toxin can be fatal.

But don't be depressed! The toxin is readily destroyed by boiling.

Specifically, a temperature of 248° Fahrenheit must be maintained at least ten minutes to kill the spores. Or using regular kitchen equipment, the poison can be destroyed by boiling foods for twenty minutes.

Having read this, don't panic and run into your kitchen to throw out all your store-bought canned goods. Actually, most if not all problems with botulism today are traceable to improper home canning—usually corn, beans, spinach and mushrooms. Fruits pose less of a hazard because of their acid content. If you are going to prepare and put up your own vegetables, learn something about the safety procedures before you do so! Get explicit instructions on how long you should cook each product before you can or jar it—or lick the spoon you just stirred it with.

There is no reason to be concerned about commercially canned foods, unless, however, you see a can bulging, or find when you open it, gas escapes or the food has an off-color or odor. The fact that virtually all of us will go through our lives without ever having to think of the possibility of botulism or any other dread food-borne disease is a tribute to the food industry and our federal food legislation when has set such high standards.

A Discourse on Chewing and Swallowing

Chewing and swallowing in a section on food safety? Yes! A Harvard University professor recently wrote a first-person article on this subject for the professional journal *Archives of Environmental Health*. We can all learn something from his story.

Our professor was having dinner at the Harvard Club in Boston. He and his group had cocktails and were enjoying a steak dinner, listening to a speaker tell a very funny story. Everyone was laughing—and eating. When the professor laughed at one punch line, he drew in a deep breath, exhaled and then stopped breathing. And he just sat there, slowly beginning to turn blue. His dinner companions stared at him and began to wonder if he was having a heart attack or a stroke. He wasn't. The last piece of steak had gone down his windpipe as he was laughing, got stuck, and now he could no longer breathe.

The fact is that you can choke to death on a morsel of food in four minutes or less. Each year, an estimated 2,500 to 4,000 United States citizens die this way, a figure that makes choking the sixth major cause of accidental death. One reason the victims die is that the onlookers often assume that he is having a heart attack and take the wrong types of steps to help.

Well, our professor survived his choking episode, but only because he knew what was happening. With all his might he exhaled the little bit of air left in his lungs and managed to cough the food out. He referred to his experience as "a bona fide brush with death."

So what are you going to do about it? First, chew your food carefully. This choking incident most often occurs in restaurants (as a matter of fact, it is referred to as a "cafe coronary"). Be particularly careful with steak, lobster, clams, roast beef and hamburger; and be even more careful if you've had a few cocktails, as it appears that alcohol dulls the gag reflex. If you are ever the victim of this problem, *do not* run off to the lavatory and assume you can take care of the problem yourself. Exhale as powerfully as you can. And try to signal for help. The best way someone can help you out—or you can help someone else if the situation is reversed—is to slap you on the back between the shoulder blades and on the upper chest, just below the throat. The point is to dislodge the piece of food.

DOLLAR-WISE DINING

In this chapter we've been dealing with approaches to eating in a modern world. We can't conclude the chapter without at least a brief discussion of what appears to be a "modern food concern" on the minds of most of us eaters: the rising cost of food.

A fractured budget does not have to mean fractured adequacy in meals. There is no Parkinson's Law that says that a food gets more and more nutritious as it becomes more and more expensive.

Stewing meat and chuck steaks contain the same amount of protein, minerals, and vitamins as sirloin or tenderloin or chops, and then, tenderizers do wonders for chewability. If you want steak, consider round tip over sirloin or porterhouse. Dried beans and peas are remarkably low-cost sources of protein and of some of the B vitamins. The most common vegetables, such as potatoes, cabbage, turnips, and squash, supply generous amounts of many nutrients. The way to economy is through planning. Clothes, time, work, leisure, vacations—all are planned in advance. Why not meals?

The cost of food certainly deserves careful thought. Upward of 35 percent of most people's income is spent on food. The typical family in the United States uses about one-half of this food money for meat, eggs, and milk. No wonder that prudent housewives plan for a day or two or even a week in advance!

Care in planning and purchasing brings big benefits. The largest losses are a result of careless, haphazard marketing. Though a dollar buys less food than it did a few years ago, if care is taken it can buy a great deal in the way of sanitation, convenience, and high nutritional quality. Domestic help is high and "out" in most homes. The housewife has many interests that keep her out of the kitchen. "Convenience foods"—well-washed, sanitized, and even partially cooked—take part of the food dollar today.

Meat is an example. It is important because of its excellent protein, and because of the B vitamins, iron, and other minerals it furnishes. It comes well-packaged, clean, and you can see what you get. To compare the cost of one kind of meat with another, and of one meat with fish or poultry, judgment must be based on the comparative nutritive quality. Low prices do not necessarily mean a saving. With some "specials" it's possible to buy high value, but other "bargains" provide mostly inedible bone, fat, and gristle.

Egg prices, too, merit thought. Did you know that the way to save is to buy medium-sized eggs when they are one-eighth cheaper than large eggs, or small eggs when they are one-fourth cheaper than large? Or did you know that grade-B eggs are wholesome and can be used to advantage for many purposes?

There are also ways to save money on milk. Milk's protein, calcium, and riboflavin are provided equally well by its many different forms: evaporated, skim and dry.

Care and common sense can cut costs and labor too. Well-selected supplies save pennies, and the pennies quickly add up to dollars. The facts are that you can buy more and more nutrition for less and less money if you plan well ahead and purchase wisely.

So there are ways to save money and still have good nutrition. Whether you're eighteen or eighty and cooking for eighteen or one, why not try these tips for cutting costs and making better meals.

General Guidelines at Home: Planning Ahead

1. Plan menus and marketing needs ahead, to ensure regular meals and thrifty use of leftovers and of seasonal and weekly specials. Keep track of the specials in your local paper. If it's practical to do so, shop around for specials.

2. Choose a variety of everyday foods to supply vitamins, minerals and other nutrients, and don't spend extra money to buy them as food supplements or as pills.

3. Let new recipes and seasonings add interest to low-cost foods.

4. Make sure your time is worth the extra price you pay for convenience foods.

5 Consider varying your old recipes. For instance, chicken or turkey cutlets can replace veal in parmesan and scallopini dishes if veal is out of the reach of your pocketbook.

General Guidelines in the Store: Looking at Labels and Buying Wisely

1. Don't shop when you are hungry! Everything begins to look good at that point.

2. Compare quantities and prices. For example, there is often a big difference in the price of two identical products, though the bottles or cans contain exactly the same quantity. Make sure your extra pennies are not just paying for a fancy package or expensive advertising. The new food labels should help you a great deal here, and may lead you to consider the "house brands" over the nationally advertised ones.

3. Be flexible. If prices for one thing are temporarily high, switch to another. For instance, if iceberg lettuce has skyrocketed in price, choose escarole, spinach, chicory or romaine. They are usually less expensive, and you get more vitamin A for your dollar too.

4. Figure cost per serving.

5. Don't be fooled by sizes and shapes. For example: two brands of one item look alike, and both cost two for twenty-nine cents, but one is an eight-ounce jar whereas the other is a nine-ounce jar. Again, read the labels.

6. Since the largest containers are usually the cheapest, buy the biggest that you can use up. Some frozen vegetables, for instance, now come in large plastic bags. They are particularly economical because you can take out what you want and store the rest.

Specific Pointers on Purchasing: Choosing Carefully

1. For protein foods: use extra cheese, peas, beans, fish and poultry, and only the economical cuts of meat.

2. For fruits and vegetables: select only what is seasonal, sound and unbruised. In cans: broken pieces are good value, food-wise and money-wise.

3. For bread and cereal: choose enriched products, save on day-old items, don't pay extra for small boxes or for sugar coating, and remember that what is baked or cooked at home is cheaper than what comes ready-to-eat.

4. For eggs: note that (1) there's no food difference between brown-shelled and white-shelled, (2) grade B is satisfactory for scrambling and for cooking foods, and (3) medium are a better buy if they are seven cents cheaper per dozen than large.

Pointers on Getting the Most Nutrient
out of the Food You Buy

1. Learn how to prepare foods in the manner which ensures you end up eating the nutrients, instead of throwing them down the sink or putting them in the garbage.

2. Take care of your vegetables. Remember that different parts of the plant have different nutrient contents. For example, leafy parts of collard greens, turnip greens, and kale have much more vitamin A than the stems. The outer leaves of lettuce are coarser than the inner tender leaves, but they have higher calcium, iron and vitamin A value, so use the outer leaves as well as the inner ones.

3. Cook your vegetables right! The best way is to cook them only until tender, in just enough water to prevent scorching. That way you'll minimize your loss of the B vitamins, vitamin C and some minerals. Use a pan with a tight-fitting lid. If you like potatoes, remember that in boiling peeled potatoes, or in whipping them afterwards if they were boiled in their skins, you lose much of the vitamin C. You keep the vitamin content high if you boil them or bake them with jackets on.

4. Don't keep foods in the freezer or on your shelves too long. Mark them with dates as you put them away. Keep canned foods cool (but not at freezing temperatures) and frozen foods *very* cool, preferably at zero degrees Fahrenheit or less.

FOUR BONUS TIPS FOR A HEALTHY DIET

1. What Is Sodium?

The Teutons waged war over it. In ancient cities the penalty for carrying it away was rather harsh—immediate decapitation or dismemberment. African wives and children in the nineteenth century were sold into slavery for it. Ancient Jews wrote laws permitting a man to divorce his wife if she did not use enough of it in food preparation.

Salt. Sodium. Whatever you want to call it, it's been around a long time. And it's been considered essential to good eating. The word has found its way into our language in many ways. Calling someone "the salt of the earth" is considered a compliment. So is indicating that someone is "worth his salt." At the medieval dinner table, he who sat "above the salt" was the honored guest. Servants and lower castes always sat "below the salt."

But despite its rich history, it seems that salt, though it does do delightful things to food, may be harmful to us if we use it in excess.

Salt occurs naturally in almost all the foods we eat. It is usually added in varying amounts in the cooking of foods and in the preservation of some foods such as ham, bacon, olives, and fish. Most Americans use far more salt on food than is actually needed—more by as much as ten to twenty times. In view of the fact that restriction of salt is an accepted and frequently useful procedure as part of the treatment of the common type of high blood pressure, it would appear to be common sense to add salt with some discretion. There is no need automatically to douse the food with salt before it is even tasted. As with everything else, use moderation. Your food will actually taste better. You will flatter your hostess by assuming that the food has been seasoned properly, and you will be forming food habits which may help maintain health.

Cutting down on salt is not a means of losing body fat. Salt contains *no* calories. But a decreased intake of salt usually results in a loss of body weight because less water will be retained in the body tissues.

Furthermore, one should always use iodized salt, thus making sure he receives enough of the important mineral iodine, which is necessary for the formation of the hormone thyroxin.

Keeping your salt intake to a moderate level is a good health idea for all of us. Don't wait until you have a problem and have to go on a low-sodium diet. Protect your health now. Animal studies have demonstrated that in certain strains of rats excess salt intake interferes with growth and raises blood pressure. And although there is no solid evidence that salt can induce hypertension in human beings, it is known that congestive heart failure can be exacerbated by high-salt levels and relieved by less dietary salt. Toxemia of pregnancy, certain types of kidney disease and hypertension can frequently be relieved by drastic reduction of salt consumption.

Furthermore, natural everyday salt is habit-forming, and many doctors would like to have less of it used in infancy and childhood so as not to form this habit. We have used sodium and salt interchangeably, but sodium is what should be reduced in our diets and salt is our major source of sodium.

2. The Low-Cholesterol School

We mentioned this topic back in chapter two in the discussion of the different types of fats which may be part of our diet. But here we want to emphasize that it's never too early—or too late—to plan meals which will tend to keep your blood cholesterol level and that of your family members low.

A few years ago there was little evidence to support the commonly accepted idea that the amount of cholesterol in the blood is related to the cholesterol of the diet. Most of the evidence showed that within a wide variation of cholesterol consumption, certainly any range found in our usual diets, the level of cholesterol in the diet did not affect the level in the blood. It is the latter value that really matters according to us in the low-cholesterol school.

However, in recent years studies have shown that these older studies were in error and that dietary cholesterol *does* influence the level in the blood. This is particularly true of the cholesterol in egg yolk.

Cholesterol from the diet is referred to as exogenous cholesterol, or "outside" cholesterol. But we also produce cholesterol, and we produce most of it in our liver and from the saturated fat in our diet. This cholesterol is called endogenous, or "inside" cholesterol. Strangely, to some extent, the less cholesterol in the diet, the more our liver makes, but it does not make enough to make up for what we omit from our diet.

Cholesterol varies in the blood from day to day, more so in some people; and those who do have a variable cholesterol may show variation by as much as 20 percent within even a few hours. Thus no one should put too much reliance on a single measurement of cholesterol in the blood, particularly if it is out of line with what was expected. An average of two or three determinations on samples of blood taken on two or three different days will give a much better idea of the real amount of cholesterol in the blood.

But there are many things involved in the development of heart and blood-vessel diseases other than an increase in blood cholesterol. So don't let what you think is a high-cholesterol amount disturb you. This is something for your doctor to interpret and advise you on.

To help lower the amount of cholesterol in your blood you should decrease the amount of saturated fat in your diet and at the same time increase the polyunsaturated fats. Follow these suggestions:

1. Use fish and poultry frequently in place of meats. The latter are both higher in fat and also higher in the saturated fats.

2. When you buy meat, choose lean cuts and trim all visible fat from your meat. Veal is low in fat.

3. Use polyunsaturated vegetable oils and spreads (soybean, corn, cottonseed oils, sunflower, and safflower, for example) in place of fats high in saturated fat such as butter.

4. Limit the number of eggs in your diet to two or three per week—but don't exclude them! (Egg yolk is the major source of cholesterol in the American diet.) As an alternative, try some of those dried or frozen egg substitutes which usually have no cholesterol.

Last, and perhaps of most importance, the level of cholesterol in the blood usually rises with gain in weight, particularly if the gain in weight is rapid. So total calorie intake with weight gain or loss is an important factor in regulating blood cholesterol. Cholesterol in the blood usually decreases with loss of weight.

3. Overly-Rich Diets and Cancer: A Possible Link

The suggestion that controlling your intake of cholesterol and saturated fat-rich foods could offer you some protection from heart disease has been gathering support for over twenty-five years. But recently, evidence from around the world suggests that you may also afford yourself some protection from certain forms of cancer by cutting back on rich food.

More than half of cancers in women and at least one-third of all cancers in men in the United States are the result of poor diets. That was the conclusion reached by Dr. Gio B. Gori, deputy director of the National Cancer Institute's Division on Cancer Cause and Prevention at a recent Senate Select Committee hearing. His comments were based on the accumulating evidence from studies of international disease patterns which strongly suggest that diet plays a major role in determining one's risks of developing such diseases as cancer of the colon, breast, ovary, uterus and prostate gland. In Japan, for example, cancers of these sites are relatively uncommon as compared to their high incidence in the U.S. Japanese generally consume significant amounts of fish, rice and vegetables as opposed to fatty meats and dairy products. Interestingly, when Japanese move to our country, within a generation they develop disease patterns similar to the American-born population, this being evidence that it is an environmental factor, possibly diet, which is responsible for the differential cancer frequency, as opposed to some genetic immunity or resistance that Japanese men and women might have.

The mechanism by which overnutrition promotes cancer is still unclear (rich diets may stimulate secretion of hormones which increase cancer risk). But what is clear is that something can be done to protect ourselves from a very mysterious group of diseases. And in addition to gaining protection from various forms of cancer, more prudent diets have the additional advantage of being good for "heart health."

The advice offered by those now studying the cancer-nutrition link is twofold:

First, we must turn to a more "prudent" diet, cutting back on cholesterol and fats, particularly saturated fats. Scientists at the American Health Foundation recommend that you consume no more than 300 milligrams of cholesterol a day, preferably much less. The fact that one egg yolk alone has about 250 milligrams of cholesterol gives you an idea of how easy it is to far exceed that limit with an egg and bacon breakfast, cheeseburger for lunch and a sizzling steak to top off the evening.

In addition to limiting eggs, include more chicken, fish and veal in your diet—and many more products of plant origin such as fruits, vegetables, cereals, grains, legumes, nuts and oils. And stay away from rich creamy desserts. For snacks, in addition to fruits and vegetables, try gelatin, water ices, sherbet, angel food cake, almond macaroons, and sponge cake.

Second, American Health Foundation's president, Dr. Ernst Wynder, strongly recommends that we fight overnutrition by encouraging the food industry to produce foods designed for better health. Specifically, he has suggested that the meat industry develop strains of animals that convert higher proportions of their feed to protein rather than fat, experimenting with new high quality vegetable protein, breeding chickens which will lay eggs low in cholesterol, and marketing products that only use egg whites. Dr. Wynder described the food industry as the "most ingenious industry of all" and noted that given the incentives, industry could develop foods commensurate with the needs of sedentary man.

You should take note of the fact that the food industry is already responding: you can now buy imitation margarine and mayonnaise with half the fat content (and calories) of the real thing. And there are a variety of egg substitutes which, although they cannot be used in baking, are excellent in recipes for french toast, omelettes, and scrambled eggs. There are ways of eating more prudently, imitating the traditional American diet but drastically reducing the amounts of fat, cholesterol and calories consumed.

What about bran and other forms of "roughage" or "fiber" as a form of "protection from cancer"? This dietary fad is the current modern-day fountain of youth, promoted by authors of best-selling books on the subject. Dr. Denis Burkitt, a surgeon who spent many of his years of medical practice in Africa, and after whom one rare form of malignancy (Burkitt's Tumor) is named, is convinced that it is the lack of dietary fiber which is a major cause of five common diseases in developed countries, among them, cancer of the colon. He is joined in this hypothesis by his colleague, Dr. Hugh Trowel, a physician.

At this point, however, the "high fiber diet" idea remains just one of many hypotheses. Americans often look for quick solutions and thus are now stuffing themselves with bran. But it's risky to attribute such a complex disease to one cause. And there are gaps in the "fiber theory," among them the fact that there is no correlation between fiber content of foods and the incidence of colon cancer in countries around the world. But there is such a correlation for fat ingestion. Perhaps people eating a great deal of bran and high-in-fiber vegetables and fruit simply have little room for fatty foods.

Whether or not it offers a direct protective effect for cancer of the colon and other diseases, bran and other crude cereals are an excellent—and delicious—contribution to a well-balanced diet.

One footnote to our commentary about a cancer-diet link: we emphasize that the basis for such a link is epidemiological—that is, based on differences in disease patterns from country to country. The link is not at this point either well established or well under-stood. For example, we know much, much more about the causal link between cigarette smoking and lung cancer and much more about the tendency for high-saturated-fat, high-cholesterol diets to predispose to heart disease. The relationship of cancer and nutrition is a new field, so few definite statements can now be made. What we are presenting here is a brief summary of our current state of knowledge, with all its gaps.

4. Alcohol and Your Health

You may think it is odd that we are including a section on alcohol as part of our discussion of good nutrition, but the fact is that for many people, alcohol accounts for a significant number of calories ingested every day. It is therefore worthwhile to look at the general subject of alcohol use and abuse—and ask the question, how much is too much?

Almost all adult Americans drink alcoholic beverages at one time or another. Some drink only on special occasions. Others drink every day—sometimes to the point of intoxication. Alcohol can be part of a pleasant relaxing situation and may actually contribute to health. But on the other hand, if it is abused it can be the cause of some very serious physical and social problems.

Alcoholic beverages were presumably discovered, rather than in-vented, in prehistoric times. Their origin is buried in antiquity, though the presence of wine and beer is well attested in archaeologi-cal records of the oldest civilizations and in the diets of the most preliterate peoples. Many earlier civilizations used alcoholic bev-erages as part of their religious observances, used as a sacred drink whereby man could incorporate the "divine" power of alcohol.

But many early civilizations, including the classic Greeks, Hebrews and Romans, used alcohol for nonreligious purposes, too. Alcoholic beverages became mandatory not only in worship and in the practice of magic and medicine, but also to solemnify formal councils, to ratify compacts and crownings, to commemorate festivals, to display hospitality and to celebrate such important life occasions as birth, initiations and marriages.

From prehistoric times until about the sixteenth century, alcoholic beverages were derived from fermentation and consisted of wines and beers containing at most about 14 percent alcohol. Then, in the fifteenth century, distillation was introduced, and more potent alcoholic beverages became popular. Suddenly, instead of beers and wines which contained from 3 to 14 percent alcohol, beverages containing up to as much as 50 percent and more alcohol could be drunk.

In addition to their mood-changing properties, the crude alcoholic beverages were undoubtedly valuable foods; this is still true of such brew as the beer of the African Bantu tribes. In many of these primitive beverages the nutrients of the raw materials, including essential vitamins and minerals, are conserved. By comparison, little of these nutrients survive in the alcoholic beverages refined by modern technology for contemporary tastes, and none is left in the products of distillation. Yet one food value remains in the distillate: the alcohol itself is a rich source of calories. Alcohol contributes about 210 Calories per ounce. Since the alcohol content of a "shot" is much less than 50 percent, a cocktail or highball usually provides between 115 and 230 Calories, depending on whether the "shot" contains one or two ounces of alcoholic ingredient.

Different Types of Alcohol?

"I'll just have some white wine" is becoming one of the more popular drink orders at American business lunches and dinners. The implication of the current swing to "lighter" drinks is that you can consume as much as you wish of wine, sweet flavored compounds such as the tequila sunrise (tequila and orange juice mixture) or "fortified" milk shakes, and that they, unlike the more classic drinks of scotch, gin or bourbon are alcoholically innocuous.

For years the rumor around France has been that the red wine produced and drunk in northern France is the cause of cirrhosis; in contrast, wines from other regions and white wines in general are widely considered to be safe for consumption in any amounts. In Spain cirrhosis has been traditionally associated with port wine—but not with sherry. Germans have long bragged that their good "liver health" was the result of the fact that they drank beer which was free from the devastating health effects of European wines.

At the base of these rumors—and the one that now is leading many Americans to have three glasses of wine instead of one martini—is the belief that whatever ill effects alcohol may have are the result of the concentration of the liquor or the various nonalcoholic components that may be included in it, as opposed to the quantity in the drink itself.

Scientific research provides no basis for such a conclusion. Ethyl alcohol, or ethanol (chemically, CH_3CH_2OH), that liquid with seemingly magical properties and the ability to induce euphoria, sedation and intoxication, is the same chemical compound no matter how it is served up. Investigations of the physical effects of alcohol ingestion confirm that it makes no difference if you are drinking wine, beer, liqueurs or distilled spirits. It is the *quantity* of alcohol consumed which is critical.

The comparison of martinis, wine and beer in terms of alcohol content may seem a bit elusive at first, but the translation of their alcoholic content to a standard base is really very simple. The alcohol content of distilled spirits, like gin, whiskey, bourbon, scotch and vodka, is expressed in terms of the proof. In the United States the proof represents twice the alcohol concentration by volume. Thus whiskey labeled "100 proof" is 50 percent alcohol, that labeled "80 proof" is 40 percent alcohol.

Table wines, carbonated or still, contain about 12 percent alcohol. Although there may be considerable variation in the final product based on the type of grape used, soil and climatic conditions, harvesting and processing procedures, there is no evidence to suggest that the alcoholic content or physiological impacts of red or white wines are different.

Fortified wines, on the other hand, usually have a concentration of 20 percent alcohol by volume, the added alcohol consisting of neutral spirits usually made from wine or brandy. Liqueurs range from 20-55 percent in alcohol content. And beers, although of different color, aroma, and flavor, are all made by fermenting carbohydrate extracted from barley malt (or rice or corn) and contain 3-6 percent alcohol (lager beer) or 4-8 percent (stout).

The comparison of three glasses (assuming 5 ounces per glass) of white wine to one martini (assuming it is 3 ounces with a 5:1 ratio of gin to vermouth) is straightforward: 15 ounces of wine x 12 percent alcohol is 1.8 ounces of pure alcohol; 2.5 ounces of gin x 40 percent alcohol plus 0.5 ounce of vermouth at 20 percent alcohol equals 1.1 ounces of pure alcohol. "Never-touch-the-hard-stuff" drinkers can easily consume considerably more booze at lunch than do those who have one traditional drink.

Alcohol's Health Effects

Given the fact that alcohol, in different forms and at various levels, has been used by man since prehistoric time, it is somewhat remarkable that the overall health effects of the drink are still somewhat unclear.

Certainly much of the confusion relates to the fact that there are so many moral and ethical questions surrounding the issue of alcohol use that scientific inquiry has been thwarted. There are some very strong personal feelings about the subject. If you are a teetotaling researcher you may start out with some different ideas and premises about the subject than if you enjoy a cocktail or two before dinner each night. Further, studies of the effects of various human drinking patterns have run into the difficult reality that people do not always tell the truth about—or perhaps they just don't remember—how much they consume. Unless you carefully measure each drink, keep track of how many you have and have about the same amount each time you drink, your responses would be only an estimate. If you drink a lot, the estimate would likely be on the low side.

The immediate effects of alcohol on the body are relatively well understood. Although the rate at which alcohol is absorbed by the bloodstream is affected by how much you drink, how fast, and what is in your stomach, alcohol is internally metabolized, or burned and broken down, at a fairly constant rate. If you drink at a rate faster than the alcohol can be metabolized, the drug accumulates in your body, resulting in higher and higher concentrations of alcohol in your blood. The larger you are, the greater the amount required to attain a given concentration of alcohol. In a 150-pound man, alcohol is metabolized at approximately the rate of one drink per hour (1.5 ounces of 40-50 percent alcohol, or a 5-ounce glass of wine or a pint of beer).

Even after the first few sips of an alcoholic beverage, there may be changes in mood and behavior; these may be due to a conditioned or learned response based on previous drinking experiences. A blood alcohol concentration of 20 mg percent to 99 mg percent (which would be the case if an average-sized man drank two or three martinis within an hour) is associated with muscular incoordination, impaired sensory function and changes in mood, personality and behavior. A concentration of 100 mg percent to 199 mg percent (three to six martinis in an hour) is associated with mental impairment, incoordination, and prolonged reaction time. More concentrated drinking has more severe effects, up to and including coma and death if alcohol is consumed at high enough doses. The legal definition of intoxication is 100 mg percent—a blood alcohol level a 150-pound man can reach by drinking five 12-ounce cans of beer, three 5-ounce glasses of wine, three 3-ounce martinis or four 8-ounce mixed highballs within one hour.

The long-term effects of alcohol drinking on health are more difficult to quantify or predict. One methodological problem here is the definition of light, moderate or heavy drinking. Some studies have been relatively conservative, classifying a person as a heavy drinker if he consumes more than 1.5 ounces of pure alcohol every day—the equivalent of 3 ounces of distilled spirits. Other definitions set the limit at 2 ounces. By *any* definition used in alcohol research, 3 ounces of pure alcohol every day—6 ounces of distilled spirits or its equivalent in wine or beer—is considered heavy drinking. (We are not dealing here with "alcoholism," a term with a variety of definitions which go beyond the amount of alcohol consumed— but rather are looking at nonalcoholic drinking patterns).

If calories are a source of concern, that reason alone is enough to be moderate about drinking—be it cocktails, beer or wine. Beyond that, a rule of thumb proposed by a nineteenth-century physician, Francis Edmund Anstie (1833-1874), is still widely accepted by those medical specialists who have extensively studied the effects of alcohol. "Anstie's limit," as it is known, states that for a 150-pound man, 1.5 ounces of absolute alcohol per day—3 ounces of whiskey, well-diluted, one-half bottle of table wine or four glasses of beer— taken with meals, will not substantially increase the risk of early death and may indeed, for some individuals, promote both physical, psychological and social health. Doubling that amount per day, that is, up to the equivalent of 6 ounces of 80 proof liquor, may or may not increase your risk of developing an alcohol-related cancer, or a liver or other type of disorder (but it will certainly have an expanding effect on your waistline). Beyond 6 ounces a day, you may be asking for trouble.

* * * * *

So those are some of the questions and concerns that go with eating in a modern world. But there is another whole topic which in recent years has probably caused more alarm about food safety than any other: food additives and pesticides. As a matter of fact, this topic is so important, a whole chapter could be written about it. And indeed one has. Read chapter five and relieve your churning stomach of any worry about "chemicals."

Chapter Five

"I Hear There Are Chemicals in Our Food"

THE "IF-IT'S-NATURAL-IT'S-GOOD" HOAX

Butylated Hydroxyanisole (BHA). Butylated Hydroxytoluene (BHT). Sodium Bisulfite. Lecithin. Xanthan Gum. If you took an inventory right now, chances are you'd find most, if not all of these "chemicals" in your kitchen. And if you'd been exposed to some of the popular anti-food additive books (for instance, *200,000 Guinea Pigs, The Poisons in Your Food, How to Live in a Poisoned World, The Chemical Feast, The Deadly Feast of Life, Food Pollution: The Violation of Our Inner Ecology, Body Pollution, Eating May be Hazardous to Your Health, The Mirage of Safety, Why Your Child is Hyperactive* and many, many others, you are probably convinced that these and similar chemicals lurking in your cupboards are laboratory-conceived villains that are out to pollute your insides and scramble the genes of the next generation.

About "Poisons" and Chemicals

But before you panic, get the facts.

First, there are no "poisons" in our food. Again, the poisons are in the pens of those who write scare books and unnecessarily stir up consumer concern. As we elaborated on in our previous book, *Panic in the Pantry*, and will look at again later in this chapter, there is overwhelming evidence that the additives used in our foods today are both safe and playing health-promoting roles. As a consumer, you are in far greater danger from plain overeating, improper food preparation and storage than from food additives whose use is carefully regulated and revised as necessary. The very, very few instances of harm from excessive or careless use of additives or from their unanticipated effects are far outweighed by their many beneficial effects.

Second, stop and think of the word "chemical." What does it mean to you? Do you think of a bubbling, foaming test tube in the hands of a mad scientist with bulging eyes and an evil smile? Many people do and thus they fear "chemicals." But in reality, *everything* in our world is made up of chemicals. And that includes you. The next time you look in a mirror what you are actually seeing is approximately 65 percent oxygen, 18 percent carbon, 10 percent hydrogen, 3 percent nitrogen, 1½ percent calcium, 1 percent phosphorus and 1½ percent gold, silver and other elements. There's also some small amount of arsenic thrown in there too (15-20 milligrams to be exact). Let's face it, you are made of chemicals!

Probably part of the concerns about "those chemicals" in our food stems from the fact that their names "sound funny." Why, some of those terms you can't even pronounce, so they must be harmful, right? "Why don't we stick to nice simple, easy-to-pronounce-food, like scrambled eggs, melon and coffee," your food-faddist friend might say. Nice and simple substances? Hardly. In an egg you'll find a long list of chemicals including ovalbumin, conalbumin, ovomucoid, lipovitellin, butyric acid, and even zeaxanthine. Try to get your faddist friend to pronounce those! And in your melon? You're getting, among other things, a dose of succinic acid, anisyl propionate, amyl acetate and malic acid, the last of which sounds particularly evil. And your steaming cup of freshly brewed coffee comes complete with an assortment of chemicals including methanol, acetaldehyde, dimethyl sulfide, diacetyl butanol and methylbutanol; and despite all of those, it's good to the last drop.

Maybe if food laws required the chemical content printed on the shell of every egg, on the rinds of all fruit, on the tops of coffee cans, and on each stalk of celery, our chemical phobia would *really* be gripping!

Third, be aware that the dichotomy being drawn today between the words "artificial" and "natural" is unrealistic. A chemical is a chemical, no matter what its source. For instance, naturally-squeezed oranges contain the chemical ascorbic acid, better known as vitamin

C. Some people might refer to this as a good-old-fashioned natural chemical, the kind you know you can trust. But they would turn their noses up at the vitamin C which was made in the laboratory, labeling it "artificial." The fact remains, however, that vitamin C— or any other specific chemical that has been synthesized by man in the laboratory—is exactly the same no matter what its original source. Vitamin C is vitamin C. "Natural" is not better!

But despite these facts, the words "natural" and "good" have just about become synonymous, and anything with artificial chemicals has become suspect. Just look at some of the products being advertised now as coming with "the mother nature seal of approval," and you can get an idea of how ridiculous the situation has become. A dairy farm claims to offer sausage without "unnatural" preservatives. A yogurt company boasts of yogurt without chemical additives (a yogurt ideal for "the natural generation"), and another major food company has organically-grown tomato juice. Even certain beverage companies, the ones which "know how we feel about beer" have "gone natural." And the butter industry is now attempting a comeback by advertising its product as "a new margarine substitute ... free of chemical additives, based on an old family recipe passed down from cow to cow."

Natural, But Deadly!

Again the idea here is that if it's natural it's got to be good. But that line of reasoning does not always follow. Under some circumstances "natural" can mean harmful and even life-threatening.

The first problem is that even natural foods deteriorate with time. Sometimes the changes they undergo result in molds and other types of growths which have been linked with cancer and other diseases. It has been shown, for instance, that some "natural" peanuts develop types of molds which produce potent cancer-causing substances (aflatoxins). Some years ago, over 100,000 turkeys in Europe died after eating moldy "natural" peanut meal, and shortly after that evidence began to indicate that ingestion of moldy nuts and grains by humans in parts of Africa was associated with an unusually high rate of liver cancer. In this country the FDA and most companies carefully examine all peanut products and have, on occasion, rejected imports which look suspicious.

It's not just peanut products which can develop these problems.

Mold growths on rye, wheat, corn and sweet potatoes have been associated with equally serious problems. Even the much glorified wheat germ can turn rancid if it is left unrefrigerated for a period of time.

The second problem is that even when they are fresh and mold-free, some natural foods can wreak havoc with animal and food health. One concern about the back-to-nature movement is that people might experiment with new vegetables, for instance, bracken fern, a tender, tasty sprout which looks much like an asparagus. Bracken fern, in all its natural glory, has been shown to contain a cancer-causing agent.

The list of natural toxins, in natural foods is long and very unappetizing. When health-food stores began to proliferate a few years ago, the Food and Drug Administration became alarmed over reports that they were selling some products which are on this "natural, but forbidden" list. For instance, sassafras roots were being offered to customers who wanted to brew some homemade "additive-free" natural tea. Unfortunately, it has been established that the active ingredient in natural sassafras (safrole) is a cancer-causing agent. The FDA seized the sassafras roots and a few other natural products (including natural seeds of apricots which were being sold as tasty treats despite the fact that they contain cyanide). It now permits only the sale of prepared sassafras tea from which all traces of safrole have been removed. (If you like sassafras tea, look at the label and check that safrole has been removed; if it is a locally-produced product, write to the manufacturer and find out if the safrole has been removed). And just as we go to press, a report has appeared in the scientific literature that mint contains a toxic, possibly cancer-causing chemical, so beware of those mint juleps!

We just want to give you a taste of the problems which can go with natural foods, and we won't elaborate on the subject here. The moral of this story is to avoid the neat dichotomy that claims that natural is safe and artificial is suspect. And when you next go tripping through the Garden of Eden, have a qualified toxicologist with you.

BUT WHAT DO THOSE FOOD CHEMICALS DO?

Some people we've talked to seem to take the attitude, "We used to get along very well without chemicals. Why don't we settle the whole question by going back to doing without them?"

Well, there are many errors in that argument.

First, agricultural chemicals have been in use for centuries. America was discovered because Columbus was searching for spices, food additives! Second, it depends on what you mean by "getting along." No serious-thinking person would wish us back to the days of famine, which is precisely what we would have without food additives—and pesticides.

Then, the good old days that we remember so nostalgically, as Will Rogers put it, "ain't what they used to be, and what's more, they probably never were." It is well within our memory that half of all the apples grown were wormy; that we cut off more of the ear of corn than we were able to cook; that we threw away a good part of every peck of potatoes because they were rotten. Our expectations of quality, in other words, are a great deal higher now than they were even a couple of decades ago. We expect every apple, every potato, every orange to be good—and it usually is.

Another important change may have gone unrecognized by the city dweller, and that is the change to the big, one-crop farm. As our population increased, it became more economical for a farmer to turn his land over to the production of one crop—for example, corn. This single-crop farming has created a banquet table for the insects who pour into the fields in such prodigious numbers that the only way to cope with them is by chemical means. If you waited for their natural enemies to catch up with these insect marauders, the crop would be destroyed and the farmer wiped out. The ultimate result would be a food shortage and very high prices.

Agricultural surpluses we need not fear. They can be regulated. We need some surplus for our own protection, and with a rapidly expanding world population for the foreseeable future, food surpluses can be put to good use.

The benefit that we derive from agricultural chemicals far outweighs the risk involved in their use. This risk is minimized by research, testing, legislation, and education. The use of chemicals involves responsibility on the part of the users. It is the same sort of responsibility that we all assume when we drive a car or, for that matter, use a pair of scissors. Unless we are willing to assume responsibility we cannot have the benefits. In this case, the benefit is in having the quantity and quality of food we need today. By to-morrow there will be more people to feed, and the need to use agri-cultural chemicals will be even greater.

Coloring Agents

But let's get specific about what additives do. Consider first the additives that add color to our food. These are most under attack by naturopaths who say they don't care what color their maraschino cherries are. Of course that's up to them, but the issue of food attractiveness is more complex. Interestingly, a scientist on a govern-ment committee studying an additive which effects the color of food admitted to being color blind! We think he should disqualify him-self.

Food is a dynamic entity. Its color, as well as other of its aspects, changes with time. Frequently a change in color can occur although the food is still fully edible and still highly nutritious. But it just doesn't look good enough to eat. Food colors can anticipate and correct for this situation.

Furthermore, food must be appealing to be eaten. That's not a conditioned response. That's a gut reaction. This is especially true for children and sick adults who often need some type of incentive to eat. But it is true for the rest of the eating population too.

And there is the fact of human nature that we like food to look "the way it should." Because of changes in weather and other factors, some foods don't look the same all year round. Butter, for instance, can differ in shade by season of the year because of the changes in the pigments in the grass on which the cow is grazing. Temperature changes can keep oranges from looking the color we expect them to look. Color additives, used in very small amounts at levels which pose no threat to our health, keep food looking its "natural" color all year round.

Preservatives

One of the other common functions additives play is that of a preservative. From the point of view of our hectic lifestyle, preser-vatives lend convenience. We don't have to shop every day for a fresh supply of food. But beyond that, preservatives are our weapon against one of our historical enemies: deterioration even before the food gets into our homes. Even today the World Health Organization estimates that 20-25 percent or more of the food supply is lost each year before it gets into consumer hands—as a result of infestation by pests and rodents and because of chemical changes. Food additives slow down deterioration considerably and, as a result, make the food supply more plentiful. Again, think of how infrequently you find a worm (or worse, half a worm) in your apple. Or a spoiled commercially canned fruit or vegetable in your pantry.

Some of the commonly used preservatives you notice on your food labels include antioxidants such as the familiar BHT and BHA. As their name implies, antioxidants retard the oxidation, usually of fats that are in food products such as crackers, cookies, or prepared cereals. Thus, they retard the development of off-flavors and give such products a longer shelf life.

Sodium propionate and sodium benzoate are other examples of preservatives. They retard or inhibit the growth of various types of organisms. Sodium propionate, for example, slows down the growth of mold on bread. This saves the consumer money because it cuts spoilage and waste. It is a perfectly harmless chemical and is added to bread only in very small amounts. Actually, it is utilized by the body, as the sodium is a mineral nutrient we need and the propionate is burned for energy.

Flavors—and Other Roles Additives Play

Flavor is an important prerequisite to a nutritious diet. No matter how loaded with protein, minerals and vitamins a food is, it will go uneaten if it doesn't please the palate. So we need flavors, but where do we find them?

There are natural sources of flavor (and many of them are included in our food supply today). But there just aren't enough to meet our needs. For instance, there is not enough natural vanilla in the whole world to flavor the ice cream we consume during a year in the United States. So we synthesize in the laboratory to come up with products which impart the same taste as the original version— but have the distinction of being available in virtually unlimited quantities. In some cases, it is misleading to call these flavors "artificial" because they are identical in chemical structure to nature's own. They just happen to be made in the laboratory.

Take a look in your kitchen, and you'll find a few more of those "nasty" chemicals which make life a little bit easier. Are you concerned about the emulsifiers in your salad dressing and chocolate milk? They are there to permit an even distribution of the globules of fat. Have you ever made your own oil and vinegar dressing at home? If so, you know how difficult it is to keep the ingredients together for very long. Emulsifiers take care of this for you. Stabilizers and thickeners (including pectins, vegetable gums and gelatins) give foods such as ice cream their uniform texture and desired consistency. And there are additives which are used to control the acidity and alkalinity in making processed foods, and accelerate the maturing and bleaching processes in bread. Still others serve to retain a food's moisture, give it light texture, maintain the clarity or firmness of a product and act as anticaking or meat-curing agents.

It is because of food additives that we have at our supermarkets today such an overwhelming variety of safe, convenient, delicious and nutritious food. Compare that variety (and the specific price tags) with what you find in so-called health-food stores.

And Additives Keep You Healthy!

And one more category of "uses." People who condemn additives forget how they make our food healthier and safer. They overlook the fact that fortification of food with vitamins C and D and iodide (additives!) have all but eliminated scurvy, rickets and goiter. And they overlook the fact that the use of nitrates and nitrites is currently the best means we have to prevent the growth of deadly botulism spores on cured meats and fish. And surprise! Those widely used antioxidants, BHT and BHA, which have been the focus of criticism in recent years, may indeed be playing another important role in *preventing* human cancer of the stomach! Some additives may prove to be public health heroes after all!

These two antioxidants, BHT and BHA, were first used in a widespread manner after 1947. Then, they were added to cod liver oil, margarine, breakfast cereals and a number of other products. What we didn't know then, but do now, is that when BHT and BHA are included in the diet of laboratory animals, there is a marked reduction in stomach cancer. And some cancer epidemiologists feel that the decline we have noticed since 1947 in the human death rate from this disease may be a result of our increased use of these additives. Indeed, our country has one of the lowest death rates from stomach cancer, followed by Australia, Canada and New Zealand. The eating habits and methods of food preservation in these countries parallel ours. European countries such as Austria and Bulgaria, for instance, where there is no widespread use of anti-oxidants in foods have far higher death rates from this form of cancer.

ARE ADDITIVES BADATIVES?

After reading some of the headlines in our national and local papers, we wouldn't blame you if you began to think so! But the answer is a firm "No!" Consider the facts about a few of the food additives which have been particularly maligned by the press.

Back to BHA and BHT

Let's pick up where we left off in the previous section, with BHA and BHT. In the 1960s there were lurid reports that these pre-servatives caused eyeless offspring in rats. Of course this finding was not confirmed in other studies. Then another researcher claimed that these chemicals when fed to pregnant laboratory animals re-sulted in abnormal behavior patterns. Again no back-up evidence could be supplied. But despite the fact that these antioxidants had a clean bill of health, one United States senator called attention to these unverified reports and announced that England had decided to ban the additives (a good way for some personal publicity). The pressure was then on here to consider similar action.

The reality of the situation, however, was that in addition to the lack of evidence about the health hazards, England had *not* banned BHA and BHT and has no intention of doing so. We tell you of this example just to show how easily scare stories can spread—without facts to support them—and how the upper levels of our government occasionally succumb to the pressure of food faddists and consumer activists.

There is no need for you to be concerned about BHA and BHT. Indeed, as we pointed out earlier, you may have cause to be grateful to them.

On Nitrates and Nitrites

"But what about those chemicals they put in meat?" some consumers have asked. Nitrates and nitrites—and the cattle growth stimulant DES. Let's look at all of them.

Occasionally you'll see a newspaper headline which claims that "bacon is the most dangerous food in your refrigerator." And maybe you recall that in the propaganda that announced the first "Food Day," bacon was listed as one of the Terrible Ten. Don't believe it. Nitrates and nitrites give certain meats and fish products a fresh red appearance and produce the traditional cured flavor. Indeed it's impossible to have cured meats such as ham and bacon without nitrites because they are a part of the curing process. Nitrite, however, does more than just add color; most important, it prevents the growth of the deadly botulism agent. We'll have our franks with nitrites!

People who are concerned about the safety of these preservative-curing agents forget that we find a great deal of nitrates—good old "natural" nitrates—in water supplies, beets, radishes, eggplant, celery, lettuce, collards and turnip greens, among other sources, and nitrite is present in significant quantity in your saliva. Spinach is a rich source of nitrate—and Popeye never seemed to complain! Some of this natural nitrate is converted inside our bodies to nitrite.

At this point, there is no evidence that nitrates and nitrites in cured products pose any hazard to human health. Certainly these chemicals should be further studied, but right now they perform a unique function and, as we've said, they are already naturally present in our diet. So don't worry about them. And if you are worried, most of the nitrites are concentrated in the saliva, not the blood or other body tissues, so get a good cuspidor and rid your body of nitrites!

DES

And then there's the beef over DES. DES is the abbreviation for diethylstilbestrol, a synthetic form of estrogen which has been used since the 1940s as a form of medication and since 1954 as a cattle growth stimulant. In 1973, DES was approved for "emergency use as a morning-after pill.

DES stimulates cattle growth, making more meat available in a shorter period of time: a 500-pound animal being treated with DES will reach a marketable weight of 1,000 pounds in thirty-five days less time using 500 pounds less feed than would an animal not receiving DES. For people who worry about meat prices—like you, for instance—that can mean a very significant savings.

"But savings or not, we don't want it in our food if it causes problems!" you are probably thinking. We couldn't agree with you more! But there is no evidence that in the rare instances DES traces show up that they cause any problems.

In 1971 there was the dramatic announcement that a small number of young women who had developed an extremely rare form of vaginal cancer were the daughters of women who had been treated with DES to prevent miscarriage. When people heard that, they panicked, and there were cries, even from one of our senators, who knows better, to "get that cancer causing chemical off the dinner table!" But again, what a great way for a little publicity.

Now look at the facts: DES is an estrogen, and all estrogens can in massive doses bring about cancer. But DES is not the only source of estrogen to which we are exposed. For instance, milk, eggs and honey have estrogen. It has been estimated that there is 1,000 times the amount of estrogen in an egg than in a serving of liver from an animal treated with DES.

And that's another point. The tiny traces of DES that were found in meat from animals were limited to their livers.

People who are worrying about traces of the estrogen DES in their beef livers are forgetting that a woman's body produces estrogen. The British science journal *Nature* estimated that it would take 500 pounds of liver containing two parts per billion of DES to be equivalent (in terms of DES quantity) to the daily production of estrogen by a reproductive-age woman. Additionally, if the woman is taking the popular birth control pills, she is taking in far more synthetic estrogen than would be found in a serving of liver with DES traces.

And consider another point before you demand that cattle raisers stop using this growth stimulant. The only evidence we've had about the dangers of DES were in the young women whose mothers had been treated during pregnancy. But these women had been treated with extraordinarily large amounts of this drug. To even come near the amount they were given in one dose, and they were given several, you would have to eat twenty-five tons of beef liver containing two parts per billion of DES.

If we went around with high powered instruments looking for traces of this and that in various foods, we'd find it. If you look hard enough, you can find anything in anything. And that's what happened in the case of DES. Detection instruments became so sensitive, they could detect traces. But that doesn't mean those traces bear any practical significance in our health.

Right now when DES is used in cattle production, it is performing a useful purpose. There is no reason to believe it is causing us any harm, and we have no cause for alarm. So eat your beef liver. It's good for you!

MSG

MSG is another food additive that has received much criticism in recent years. Contrary to popular opinion, it does not stand for Mighty Suspicious Goods, but rather for monosodium glutamate. The next time you hear someone complain about this "nasty artificial food additive," remind them where much of our MSG comes from: Nature's own sugar beet, for sugar beets are one of the main sources from which MSG is made. It is simply the sodium salt of a common amino acid, a constituent of all protein, and is formed in the body whenever protein is eaten. Nothing could be more natural.

But you'll continue to hear some strange stories about MSG. Critics say it is the underlying cause of the "Chinese restaurant syndrome" experienced by some people after eating soy sauce, imported mushrooms, duck sauce—or maybe some other food containing MSG. Perhaps a few people do have adverse reactions to this ancient food flavor enhancer, much the way other individuals react adversely to eating strawberries or shrimp. But it is hardly grounds to condemn a very popular additive used as a flavor enhancer.

Then there are the claims of the single researcher who has injected massive doses of MSG into newborn mice and a single monkey and noted brain damage. Had this researcher injected almost any substance the results might have been similar. But because of the public upheaval related to the publicity given this experiment, baby-food manufacturers felt the pressure and voluntarily removed MSG from their products.

If you enjoy sprinkling MSG on your steak or burgers before you broil them, continue doing so. You have nothing to worry about.

Sweet and Dangerous?

But what about artificial sweeteners? Are they safe? And if they are, why has there been so much commotion about them in the last ten years?

Consider cyclamate, a chemical that will surely go down in the food additive hall of fame.

It was banned in 1969, after over eighteen years of use, because in one study of 240 rats eating a complex mixture which happend to include cyclamate, 8 of those at the highest dose levels developed a form of bladder cancer.

Why were they banned on the basis of such meager evidence? A few vocal so-called consumer advocates publicly, but without facts, raised questions about the sweetener during the fall of 1969. When the results of this one laboratory experiment became known, public concern was at its peak and the secretary of Health, Education and Welfare was under pressure to act.

Actually, given the results of that one study, the fate of cyclamate was inevitable because a certain very controversial piece of legislation known as the "Delaney Clause" requires that any food additive which has been shown to cause cancer in animals—even in just one experiment and even if at incredibly high dose levels—must be removed from the food supply.

Now, a number of years later, both legislators and food scientists looking back on the banning of cyclamates are realizing it was probably a mistake. Subsequent studies all over the world have shown the sweetener to be safe. Indeed, one major manufacturer of cyclamate, armed with volumes of post-1969 evidence, tried to get the FDA to change its mind. But it didn't. Why? Primarily because it's rather difficult to explain to the American public why something is harmful enough to be precipitously banned in 1969, and then is "okay" again in the late 1970s. But our guess is that cyclamates will be back, and we think they should be! At the time of this writing, a leading manufacturer of cyclamates in the cyclomate days, is taking the matter to court, demanding a new trial.

And saccharin? At the time of this writing, the ultimate fate of this sweetener is unknown. In March of 1977, preliminary results of a Canadian study were made known and the FDA announced its intention to ban it. The Canadian study (which noted urinary tumors in animals fed the equivalent of 1200 bottles of diet soda a day while in their mothers' uteri *and* during their own entire life-times) was enough to lead to a banning because of the Delaney Clause. This was in spite of the fact that saccharin has a safe history of use by humans for the past eighty years (studies of diabetics who used large amounts of the sweetener for up to twenty-five years reveal no unusual excess in cancer incidence).

In June of 1977, the press carried reports of another Canadian study, one which allegedly found that the incidence of bladder cancer was higher among saccharin users. The results of this study were not consistent with at least eight other epidemiological studies under-taken by prominent scientists from Harvard, Oxford, Johns Hopkins and elsewhere. Indeed, all of the previous epidemiological investi-gations about the possible role of saccharin in bladder cancer etiol-ogy, which involved over 60,000 persons, showed no adverse effects from saccharin use. The new Canadian Study did show a 60 percent increased risk of cancer in males—but it also showed a 40 percent decreased risk for females. Given that it is highly unlikely that saccharin has a "sex specific effect" (there is no known example of a factor which causes cancer in humans of one sex and not in the other), there is reason to doubt these results.

We have learned a great deal from the cyclamate and saccharin sagas: it is not useful or intelligent to panic about a food or a food additive on the basis of one random report or one unverified ex-periment. And we know now that having such an arbitrary law as the Delaney Clause which does not allow scientific discretion is not useful either. (See our specific comments about the Delaney Clause later in this chapter). Anyone can claim anything they want about a food. But does that mean we should immediately accept it, jump up and ban it? Of course not. You should keep that point in mind the next time you see a food additive scare story in the paper. Don't be taken in by the huffing and puffing of one or two individuals. Wait until you hear what our country's respected medical and scientific authorities and organizations have to say first.

Red 2

Until recently one of the most widely used coloring agents, Red 2, found itself under fire when a few outspoken, but not parti-cularly well-informed, individuals claimed that it caused cancer and/or birth defects in animals. You shouldn't be surprised at this point that these were the same individuals and the same "interest" groups as before who were involved in the questions raised about nitrates, nitrites, DES, etc. It was just that Red 2 provided a new target for their complaints, another opportunity for publicity and to massage their egos.

In early 1976, the "consumer advocates" were again successful, and the dye was banned. At the time of the banning, the tests done on the dye could be boiled down to two categories: one positive test (performed in Russia) and dozens of negative tests. Perhaps the ultimate shortcoming of Red Dye #2 was that it had a "funny sounding chemical name": trisodium salt of 1-(4-sulfo-1-naphthylazo) 2 naphthol-3, 6 disulfonic acid.

Additives and Hyperactive Children?

One of the more encompassing charges made about food additives in general, and color additives in particular, has been made by Dr. Benjamin Feingold, recently retired as an allergist, of the Kaiser-Permanente Medical Center in San Francisco.

He has claimed that food additives are a major cause of hyperkinesis (a behavioral disorder which causes children to be overactive, impulsive, with short attention spans that interfere with their learning ability). It is interesting to note, however, that, to our knowledge, Dr. Feingold has never published in detail a single paper in the recognized medical literature so that other physicians and scientists could evaluate his theories with his evidence. Instead, he decided to make his "findings" public through a popular book (*Why Your Child is Hyperactive*) and via television talk shows.

Do food additives make children hyperactive? Authorities who have looked into this have concluded "no." The special advisory committee convened by the Nutrition Foundation noted that "no controlled studies have demonstrated that hyperkinesis is related to the ingestion of food additives . . . the claim that hyperactive children improve significantly on a diet that is free . . . of food additives has not been confirmed." Since then, carefully conducted and well-controlled studies at the University of Wisconsin have provided no facts to support the Feingold hypothesis—or dream.

Interestingly enough, it wasn't just the professional press which did not receive Dr. Feingold's theories well. The *Library Review* noted that Dr. Feingold's book on the subject "fails to answer satisfactorily the question posed in its title for a number of reasons. . . . The work is poorly written, lacks references and documentation and is badly organized."

But again, many radio and TV shows ran series based on Dr. Feingold's idea, and parents panicked, rushing to health-food-land to avoid artificial colors. This panic was another example of what can follow the public announcement or random, unconfirmed conclusions. Shouldn't we have more than a few testimonials from just one researcher before we report something as a fact?

FLIES, MOSQUITOES, WORMS, BUGS AND PESTICIDES

"If the use of pesticides in the United States were to be completely banned, crop losses would probably soar to 50 percent and food prices would increase four to fivefold." That was the conclusion reached by Dr. Norman E. Borlaug who won a Nobel Prize for his work in developing new strains of wheat. A similar conclusion has been reached by anyone who has looked scientifically into the question of pesticide use.

We need pesticides to keep our crop level high and wastage at a minimum. For instance, potatoes are subject to attack by at least 200 insects and disease-producing agents. In the nine years after organic pesticides were introduced, the average yield of potatoes per acre was increased by 90 percent. Furthermore, the use of pesticides to eliminate flies, mosquitoes and intestinal parasites has improved pork and beef production and increased milk output. Supernaturalist Robert Rodale recommended that we "pick the bugs off potato plants," but the reality is that without pesticides every second or third potato and tomato would be lost and oranges and grapefruit would be curiosities.

Obviously, the main health value of pesticides is in raising food and preventing the possibility of malnutrition while keeping prices low. But according to Dr. Russell S. Adams, from the soil science department of the University of Minnesota, even with agricultural chemicals, insects and weeds still produce losses averaging about 50 percent of the potential U.S. strawberry crop, 30 percent of our potential potato and corn crop, 26 percent of our wheat crop and 19 percent of our apple crop. (These figures come from the USDA Agricultural Handbook.)

Critics of agriculture, Dr. Adams points out, have argued that human labor could replace the need for pesticides. Certainly the use of herbicides and to a much lesser extent, fungicides and insecticides, have some labor-saving component. However, to control these pests without pesticides and machinery would require tremendous inputs of additional labor. Modern high-speed cultivators are dependent to a considerable extent upon herbicides to control weeds within the row. If we depended on labor alone, some have estimated that it would require 17.7 million people working for six weeks to remove all the weeds from the U.S. cornfields. Assuming people worked a forty-eight-hour week and were paid $3.00 an hour, this would be equal to 115 percent of the value of the entire U.S. corn crop in 1973, or 31 percent of the entire U.S. agricultural production that year. At this cost, many foods would become prohibitively expensive.

It is recognized, of course, that proper controls must be vigilantly applied. And many steps have been taken. You needn't worry about getting harmful residues in your food. Our major food processors carefully train fieldmen to supervise growers, to oversee application of pesticides and to ensure the elapse of an appropriate amount of time between application and harvest. Both in the field and at the processing plant, samples are analyzed so that residues are below the tolerance level both before and after processing.

Much of the consumer concern about pesticides stems from a worry about how much of the pesticides remains on the food when it reaches the table. Happily, FDA studies on the American diet from market basket food samples continue to show that the amounts of residues present were not important from the health standpoint. What is more, the residues have decreased from levels found a few years ago.

The idea behind market basket or grocery bag food studies is to give scientists samples of food, which are as much like the diet we eat as possible, to test for insecticides.

The first step is for workers to go out to supermarkets in different cities across the country. These workers buy enough groceries to feed the biggest eater in the country. It will probably be no news to anyone who has watched a teen-ager raid the refrigerator that nobody eats more than a hungry teen-age boy! The scientists choose items in their shopping which would make up a good diet for him. Then it is back to the laboratory with the samples to detect any residues.

If harmful amounts of any residues got into our foods, this kind of total diet study would pick them up. The Food and Drug Administration would then put a quick stop to it by seizing dangerous foods.

As further insurance, government laboratories also test separate samples of foods for pesticide levels.   Last year over 30,000 pieces of raw foods were tested in this way.

Tests used for detecting residues from insect sprays, weed killers, and fungus destroyers get better and better each year. Even with improved methods, scientists find that actual residue levels in foods are decreasing. Ironically, the FDA and other agencies believe that many cases of the traces of pesticides that do appear are there not from farmer but from roadside weed control and insect control measures for health and forest protection.

The real danger from these chemicals is not in the tiny amounts which are found in some foods. The real hazard is that insecticides and other household chemicals are often left where small children can reach them in the home.

We must stop the tragic and needless poisoning of small children who eat or drink carelessly stored substances such as insecticides. Toddlers love to taste all sorts of things. The wise mother knows that garden sprays, window cleaners, bleaches, and strong cleaning solutions should be kept out of sight and reach.

Any compound can be toxic if too much of it gets into the body. In fact, the majority of fatal as well as less serious poisoning accidents in this country are from the misuse of fairly nonpoisonous materials. A sad example of this was front-page news only a few years ago. Infants were accidentally poisoned by salt in high amounts being used instead of sugar in their formulas.

Insect spray levels in foods are carefully policed by the Food and Drug Administration. The responsibility for the care and control of pesticides in the home is ours. Americans have a long way to go in improving home safety records. A good step in this direction would be for everyone who reads this book to make sure that all household chemicals are out of the reach of those too young to know their dangers.

Pesticides Banned

In November 1959, large quantities of cranberries were recalled because they had been sprayed with the "cancer-causing agent" aminotriazole. On Thanksgiving Day that year, many people were concerned enough about all cranberry sauce that they omitted the item from their menu (but, of course, many lit up cigarettes after their cranberryless meal).

In 1962 Rachael Carson produced a shock wave by publishing the book *Silent Spring*. Many regard this book as an eloquent and emotional plea to protect wildlife, especially songbirds, against being poisoned by sprays. Actually, as pointed out by Professor Thomas H. Jukes from the Department of Medical Physics at Berkeley, the main thrust of the book is the concept that pesticide residues in our foods will give us cancer and other degenerative diseases. *Silent Spring* soon became the bible of environmentalists and the health-food movements, and has remained in this position ever since—despite the fact that the pages of that work are loaded with inaccuracies, exaggerations and downright untruths (such as the statement that "the American robin is on the verge of extinction," written at the time when this species was undergoing a population explosion because of its expansion of habitat in surburban areas). But the greatest failing of the book is its careful omission of any mention of the fact that DDT has saved more human lives and prevented more diseases than any chemical in history.

Since the cranberry scare and publication of *Silent Spring*, many other pesticides have been indicted as human cancer risks: aldrin and dieldrin have been banned on the grounds that they cause liver tumors in mice. In making the decision that aldrin and dieldrin were "imminent hazards," the Environmental Protection Agency overlooked the facts that phenobarbitol, a widely-used drug which is taken in significantly higher doses than are the traces of pesticides that may show up in food, also causes liver tumors; that the mouse is generally considered to be an inappropriate test model for the purpose of predicting carcinogenic response in man; that aldrin and dieldrin did not cause cancer in other animals, for instance, the dog; and that men who had worked closely with these chemicals for many years, being exposed to levels many hundred times those of the general population, did not have unusually high rates of any form of cancer.

The most immediate effect of the banning of pesticides in this country is an increase in the price of food following an inevitable cutback on the availability of produce. But environmental regulations in this country can create serious health problems abroad, especially in the underdeveloped nations.

The scientist who heads the United Nations' crop protection program says that American pesticide regulations are making it impossible for underdeveloped nations to get enough agricultural chemicals. Dr. William Furtick, chief of Plant Protection Services for the UN's Food and Agricultural Organization (FAO) has recently emphasized the need for more pesticides and more pesticide diversification in developing countries.

Increased use of pesticides will have to be a "major ingredient" in any developing-world agricultural expansion. But developing nations depend on the highly industrialized nations for these products and are therefore, in his words, "at the mercy of regulatory fads." Pesticide manufacturers whose products are banned or severely restricted in the U.S. or other developed countries aren't likely to manufacture those banned products for the smaller "third world" market only.

While crop losses to pests are substantial here, such losses can be absolutely staggering in underdeveloped nations. FAO and other experts estimate that up to half the world's total food supply in a given year is consumed or destroyed by pests and plant diseases, and even after a "successful" harvest, losses in storage can be disastrous. In India, for example, losses of *stored* grains are often up to 70 percent.

"Toxic" vs. Hazard

One of the favorite words food faddists use in their fight against additives is "toxic." It *is* a rather scary word. Certainly none of us wants to eat toxic food. But the fact remains that many, many foods that we eat every day have chemicals that we know are toxic. But don't get alarmed!

For instance, we mentioned that salt can be toxic if consumed in large amounts. You might have already known or suspected that. But did you know that our natural potato also has a toxic substance or two in it—specifically solanine, the very chemical which is found in the foliage of the deadly nightshade. By consuming an average of 119 pounds of potatoes a year, we take into our system about 9,700 milligrams of the toxin, solanine, enough to kill a horse. But it doesn't bother us. Consider another example: lima beans, which we consume on the average of 1.85 pounds per year. Lima beans contain hydrogen cyanide (which was one of the nazis' favorite suicide potions). And fruits, vegetables, cereal products, meats and dairy products all have traces of the toxic chemical arsenic.

The list of foods with one or more "toxic" substances in them is long. But we're not telling you this to get you more agitated than you already may be. The point is that there is a vast difference between the words "toxic" and "hazardous." The toxicity of a substance is its intrinsic capacity to produce injury when tested by itself, usually in large amounts. A hazard, on the other hand, is the capacity of a substance to produce injury under the circumstances of exposure.

In other words, there is a toxic substance or two in lima beans and potatoes—and if you were to remove this substance and eat it alone and in quantity you'd get sick. You might even die. But given the circumstances under which we eat potatoes and lima beans there is no cause for concern. Why? Because the levels in these products are so low they don't bother us. These toxic substances don't "store themselves up" to become a hazard. And because we eat so many other chemicals—natural and otherwise—in foods, they may even offset each other.

Now think about food additives. Yes, if you isolate a certain food additive and feed it in high doses to an animal it might be hazardous. But in the normal usage in food, it, like the toxic substances in vegetables and other "normal" foods, presents no problem. The same reasoning applies in the case of pesticides.

THE DELANEY CLAUSE

Much of the pandemonium recently about food additives and pesticide residues is the result of the existence of a piece of legislation that states, "No additive shall be deemed to be safe if it is found to induce cancer when ingested by man or animal, or if it is found, after tests which are appropriate for the evaluation of the safety of food additives, to induce cancer in man or animals. . . ." The law was passed in the final hours of Congressional debate about the 1958 food additives amendment. One of the many nonscientists testifying in favor of the clause was health faddist Gloria Swanson, somewhat better known at that time for her dramatic abilities.

At the time of its introduction, the law was considered by many to be an undesirable supplement to an already comprehensive food additive regulatory system. But in the twenty years since it has become law, the limitations of the so-called anticancer clause have come clearly into focus. It is worth taking the time here to point out some of the problems with the clause—and why we feel it should be deleted.*

Delete the Delaney Clause!

President Ulysses S. Grant, in his inaugural address in 1869, set forth a common sense-based philosophy about the dilemma of unnecessary, irrelevant unconstructive laws: "I know of no method," he said, "to secure the repeal of a bad or obnoxious law so effective as its stringent execution." In early March of 1977, with the FDA's announced intention to ban the artificial sweetener saccharin, President Grant's words became noticeably applicable to the Delaney Clause.

The fact that the future of saccharin was suddenly in jeopardy brought into focus for many Americans—for the first time—the question of how we determine what is and is not safe for human consumption. In the past, food safety issues did not always seem fully relevant to everyday meal planning and the majority opinions were: "So what if they ban the chemical that makes maraschino cherries red? We can live without it." "Who needs food colors anyway?" "If DES is banned, beef will cost a few cents more a pound . . . so what?"

But with saccharin, it was a different story. When applied literally and strictly, as Grant predicted, the law in question—the Delaney Clause of the 1958 Food Additives amendment—eventually hit a nerve.

The Delaney Clause is an example of how the real spirit of law can be thwarted by personal politics and unrestrained advocacy. The clause has good intentions—after all, no one in his right mind would want to add cancer-causing chemicals to our food supply. Indeed, because of its underlying good intentions, the clause has great appeal

---

*An alternative suggestion we have made is that the clause be *strengthened*, to include not only artificial food additives—but all chemicals, no matter what their origin—which cause not just cancer but any disease or deformity in any laboratory animal. Given, then, that almost all foods would be eligible for a ban, the absurdity of the law would become even more apparent.

to common sense and emotions of the average person. But in practical terms—and in dealing with the realities of what causes human cancer—the Delaney Clause is at best scientifically naive, and at worst dangerously misleading. It is a law based on a highly emotionally-charged fear of a devastating disease, cancer, and it is an underlying cause of another serious and widespread ailment—cancerphobia.

We will only touch on seven main limitations of the clause.

First, the Delaney Clause is an arbitrary, inflexible statute which requires the banning of a food additive on the basis of one or a limited number of laboratory animal experiments, even though those experiments may contradict the general knowledge about the carcinogenicity of that substance. The lack of discretion in the Delaney Clause contrasts sharply with that afforded in other sections of the food and drug law which sets tolerances for "poisonous or deleterious substances" whose addition cannot be avoided.

Those defending the position that the addition of the adjective "appropriate" to describe tests capable of invoking the clause does allow discretion, overlook the fact that the mere existence of the clause and the awareness that one set of positive results in a cancer experiment is enough to lead to a banning, creates an atmosphere of fear and urgency where decisions are based not on facts but on what a chemical might possibly do.

Judgments on the relative safety of environmental chemicals are often difficult to make. It is unrealistic, unsophisticated and untenable in the world of carcinogenesis where a multitude of variables may be involved in causation.

Second, the Delaney Clause relies heavily on the assumption that animal experiments are excellent predictors of the cancer-causing potential of a chemical in man. Indeed, proponents of the clause often point out that all chemicals that cause cancer in man cause cancer in animals, the implicit conclusion being, then, that mice are little men. While it is true that most, but not all, known human carcinogens are cancer-causing agents in laboratory animals (an exception here would be the known human bladder carcinogen, beta-napthylamine which does not have a cancer-causing impact on the bladders of rats or mice), *the opposite is not true*—all animal carcinogens are not human carcinogens. For example, drugs such as sodium penicillin and phenobarbitol are known animal carcinogens but have no known cancer-causing effect in humans. If the philosophy of the Delaney Clause were applied to the oral contraceptive—which contains a synthetic estrogen—The Pill would never have been approved, given that all estrogens, natural or otherwise, have carcinogenic properties.

There is no doubt that animal experimentation plays a critical role in chemical safety evaluation. We are not suggesting that we rely solely on evidence of human experience with a substance. Nor are we proposing that we return to the early century study protocol of Dr. Harvey Wiley who fed human volunteers—the so-called Poison Squad—high doses of food additives to see how they reacted. Epidemiology does have its limitations, primary among them that it takes five, ten, twenty, or more years for some human carcinogens to make known their deadly characteristics. But we should not be guided by a law which assumes that the laboratory animal fed excessively high doses is an infallible predictor for man. Again, this relates back to Delaney Clause limitation number one—inflexibility.

Animal experiments need to be interpreted, put in proper perspective. Possible individual species or strain susceptibility must be taken into account, as well as other unique circumstances that may have been responsible for whatever positive results may have appeared.

If a food additive, when ingested in large amounts by a group of rats, led to an increased incidence of malignant tumors of the bladder, liver or other organ, we think the results are worth noting. But that observation is certainly not enough to warrant the condemnation of that chemical. Instead, such an observation should stimulate similar tests on other animals. When a series of different tests on different animals are in, the scientific decision-making process could begin: Were the results consistent—or somewhat consistent? At the very least, did the chemical have a carcinogenic effect in more than one species? What about a dose-response relationship? Did the incidence of tumors increase as the dosage of the chemical was increased? Does the chemical being evaluated have any characteristics that might lead one to suspect it is carcinogenic? Are there specific factors which promote or inhibit the carcinogenic effect of this substance in a laboratory animal? Is there any human epidemiological evidence available on the substance which would support or fail to support the laboratory findings? Certainly years of safe use by humans should carry more weight than one limited animal evaluation. The answers to some, if not all, of these questions may provide a basis for sound, scientific decision-making. There can be no set rules—any more than there are set rules in judging the relative safety of drugs. The data provided by laboratory experimentation should provide one input, an important input, into a complex evaluation procedure.

Third, the Delaney Clause, and we might add the spirit of regulatory guidelines outside the food additive area which appear to be based on the general philosophy of the Delaney Clause, is unrealistic and, indeed, anachronistic in that it assumes that if large amounts of a substance induce cancer in animals or humans, then even trace amounts, minute quantities, could also be carcinogenic.

This zero tolerance principle is, as is the case with the clause in general, deceptively simple and emotionally appealing. "Why take the chance?" is the common reasoning. "A little bit of a carcinogen might cause a little bit of cancer, so we should eliminate our exposure to all of it." Such a statement ignores scientific knowledge and capabilities.

All known human cancer-causing agents have some "dose response" curve. Individuals smoking two cigarettes a day for ten or more years show no appreciable increase in mortality from lung cancer. Those smoking ten, fifteen, twenty, thirty or more cigarettes a day show an increasing tendency to die from lung cancer. Individuals who spend a great deal of time in the direct sunlight, particularly if they are fair-skinned, have a high probability of developing skin cancer sometime in their lives. But the fairest of all individuals spending limited time in the sun is highly unlikely to develop a sun-induced skin cancer.

Again, proponents of the clause will claim: "We do not know how to establish with any assurance at all a safe dose in man's food for a cancer-producing substance." That is just another way of saying we can't prove something is safe—which is true. In setting guidelines for chemical exposure—whether in food, the workplace or elsewhere— what we are looking for are levels which by all reasonable standards apparently cause no harm.

Fourth, and related to the problems of the zero tolerance principle, the Delaney Clause is particularly unacceptable today, given the sophisticated means we have of detecting minute levels of a substance. This limitation of the clause will become increasingly apparent with the growing sophistication of analytical chemistry. At the time the law was enacted, toxicologists were able to detect adulteration on the order of one part per million. Today sensitivities are below one part per billion, well on their way to parts per trillion.

Fifth, the clause is inconsistent in that it only applies to artificially produced food additives. It seems to prefer naturally occurring carcinogens to man-made ones. Thus, you have a situation where saccharin, cyclamates or red dye could be banned as cancer-causing agents, yet it is well-known that naturally occurring carcinogens surround us. Safrole, a component of some essential oils and several spices, causes liver tumors in rats, and indeed it was this factor which led to its banning as an artificial food additive. Aflatoxins, probably the most potent chemical inducers of liver cancer, are made by molds which grow naturally on such products as peanuts and wheat, but the Delaney Clause is not interested in them. Estrogens, the source of concern in discussions about the safety of DES in raising cattle, are widely found in nature's own products—wheat, soybeans, green leaves, vegetable oil, even wheat germ, the standby of most food faddists—all containing far more estrogenic activity than has ever been found in liver from estrogen-treated cattle.

Sixth, the Delaney Clause is blind to the concept of benefit and risk. If nitrites are shown to cause cancer in ducks, they are vulnerable to the effects of the anticancer clause; they could be banned even though they are considered essential for protecting us from the deadly botulism toxin in cured meats. But cured meats only account for about 15 percent of the nitrite content of our diet, the rest of the nitrite—85 percent of the total—comes from radishes, celery, spinach and other vegetables. Should they be banned from our diets?

Seventh, and probably the most devastating impact of the Delaney Clause, is the fact that it acts as a distractionary, divisive factor in the ongoing pursuit of knowledge about what does cause cancer.

By stimulating almost weekly reports about allegedly "cancer-causing" agents in the food supply, the Delaney Clause is serving to intensify cancerphobia in America, distracting consumers from proven human cancer threats like cigarette smoking. With the banning of saccharin, individuals began to dwell on the possibility that the artificial sweetener could cause bladder cancer. Sadly, the majority of Americans aren't even aware that one-third of U.S. bladder cancer is directly induced by cigarette smoking.

The clause has caused the diversion of limited research monies to evaluate and reevaluate food additives which have never been linked to human cancer when these funds could be more beneficially invested in a research area which shows real promise of pay-off, specifically, the epidermiological link between diet—general food selection, not additives—and cancer of the breast, colon, prostate and uterus.

The existence of the Delaney Clause has had an unsettling effect on consumer confidence in the FDA, causing that agency to take action which did not have consumer support. The saccharin example is the most vivid one here, there being something ironic about the fact that the day after our government health agency informed us that saccharin may be a cancer threat, consumers flocked to the stores to clean out supplies.

And the clause has been divisive in creating two camps—the image of the money-grubbing industry types who don't care what is put in their foods versus the people-loving consumer activists who are dedicated to protecting all of us. The dichotomy is an absurd one. We all want our food to be safe. We also want it to be available in quantity, to be as inexpensive, convenient and attractive as possible. Polarization, and that is what the Delaney Clause has created in its twenty years of existence, is not the means to that end.

In conclusion, the Delaney Clause should be deleted. Alternatively, it could be modified. But in our opinion, modification would, for all practical purposes, be the same as deletion, although perhaps more politically palatable, since modification in practically any way would neutralize the clause's main flaw: arbitrariness.

The clause is a regulatory crutch which presents an impractical impediment to sensible decision-making. We need rational, politically blind, scientifically based laws which take into account consumer wants and needs to ensure the safety and availability of a wide variety of drugs and foods. We *do* need a federal regulatory system to ensure that environmental chemicals are by the current standards safe. In the absence of the Delaney Clause, the FDA would still have full power to regulate food safety. No additional regulation is necessary. There *are* legitimate instances in which government agencies have acted decisively and correctly. For example, the FDA has refused to approve laetrile which has been repeatedly shown to be ineffective in the prevention or treatment of cancer. It is our hope that the current saccharin flap has dealt a mortal wound to the Delaney Clause, one which will accelerate our entrance into an age of new and more reasonable approaches to evaluating the chemicals in our lives.

Chapter Six
But What About . . .

NUTRITION DURING PREGNANCY

Well, what about nutrition during pregnancy? Should you wait until you find out conception has occurred and then follow the old (and misleading) adage "a pregnant woman should eat heartily because she is eating for two," usually interpreted as for two adults? No, not really.

First, from the medical point of view, it's a good idea to evaluate carefully your diet before pregnancy occurs. Why? Because the first two or three weeks after conception is a critical time in the growth of the embryo, and since this is a period during which most women don't know they are pregnant, it's better to be nutritionally prepared ahead of time.

Second, it is not wise to approach pregnancy meal-planning with the idea that you are eating for two—especially if it's two adults you have in mind. Some women when they learn they are pregnant assume that they can eat as much as they like during those special months, imagining pregnancy as a temporary reprieve from an ongoing worry about weight problems. Not so. As a matter of fact, for many pregnant women the concern about gaining extra pounds too quickly is a very serious one.

You might initially be surprised to learn that a woman during her early pregnancy weeks needs very few if any extra calories and later needs only about 200-300 more Calories each day than she normally does. That might appear to you to be an unreasonably small addition, but the fact is that fetal growth, until the last three months of the pregnancy, is relatively small, and thus the "extra" calorie needs are minimal. The growing fetus does not need an exorbitant number of calories. And neither does the prospective mother. While it is obvious that pregnancy is no time to go on a crash diet, excessive calorie intake and the inevitable extra pounds that will follow are not only unnecessary, but may well pose a risk to both the health of the baby and mother.

If you are pregnant, your physician will set guidelines on how much weight gain is permissible for you, but for most women about twenty-two to twenty-seven pounds over the full course of pregnancy is ideal.

What about the type of diet? Again, there may be some special individual requirements, but generally the following foods might well be included each day during the first half of pregnancy. This daily diet for the average woman will supply about 2,000 Calories and 70 to 80 grams of protein:

1-2 glasses of milk in some form
1-2 servings of meat, fish, or poultry
1 serving of citrus fruit
1-2 servings of other fruits
2 or more servings of vegetables, one of which should be dark green or deep yellow
4 or more servings of breads and cereals—enriched or whole grain.

In the second half of pregnancy one should expect to gain from fifteen to twenty pounds. It is during this period that the fetus starts growing, maternal blood volume increases, and other physiological changes take place. As a result you need more protein (about 80-100 grams a day) and can raise your Calorie intake by some 300.

To the food amounts outlined for the first half, add the following: Another glass of milk (nonfat if you are having trouble with your weight), and another serving of citrus fruit, of leafy, green vegetable, and of meat, fish, or poultry.

Your physician is the one to adapt this general guide to your individual weight and food needs during pregnancy. So again, take the doctor's advice to ensure your own healthy pregnancy!

Are there any special needs you should keep in mind during pregnancy, other than the increase in protein we have already mentioned? Your doctor will also give you advice on this, but generally the growth in fetal tissues and the changes occurring in your body require also an increase in folic acid, most of the other B vitamins, vitamin C and minerals such as iron, calcium, phosphorus, iodide, fluoride and magnesium. Most of these needs can be met by making sure you balance your diet, eating a variety of foods within the categories listed above. If you follow this dietary pattern, drink fluoridated water and choose milk that has been fortified with vitamin D (if skimmed milk, fortification with vitamins A and D), most all your nutrients for good health during pregnancy can be derived from your meals. The two exceptions might be iron and folic acid since it is difficult to get these in generous amounts through food alone. Your doctor may well prescribe a supplement to supply them.

Youthful Pregnancy

It is generally accepted that a healthy, well-nourished woman is more likely to have a healthy, full-term baby than is an undernourished, sickly one.

In this country we have long been aware of the importance of proper nutrition, not only during pregnancy, but before it as well. The importance of this cannot be overemphasized. But despite the extensiveness of our knowledge and widespread acceptance of the importance of nutritional principles, young prospective mothers—generally those of high-school age—still remain at risk of nutritional problems.

As we mentioned above, pregnancy, even in physically mature women, leads to additional and new nutritional needs. When these demands of pregnancy coincide with the nutritional demands of adolescence, the health of both the mother and child may suffer. In short, a pregnant adolescent has undertaken the development of another human being before her own body is mature.

Many teen-age women, as a result of their eating habits and/or patterns, may have nutritional deficiencies. Often they are unaware of the effects of poor nutrition. Hamburgers and Cokes by themselves, often a routine diet, will not meet their nutrition needs in the critical years. This diet is indeed inadequate when considered in view of the additional burdens of pregnancy. A young girl—seventeen years or younger—who is in less than the best of health when she becomes pregnant, is borrowing trouble for herself and lending it to the child she carries. She should seek the counsel of a physician as soon as she suspects that she is pregnant and follow his advice—which generally will emphasize the importance of eating a variety of foods based around the Basic Four Food Groups and possibly routine vitamin and mineral supplements—in order to optimize her chances for her own good health and a successful childbirth.

BREAST-FEEDING

Women who are disappointed that they can't take advantage of pregnancy to stock up on extra calories may enjoy breast-feeding, or lactation, better.

Generally there is a significant increase in the number of Calories a breast-feeding woman needs — some 500 to 1,000 above her normal intake. This assumes, of course, that you are resuming your normal range of activities plus the care of a child. With breast-feeding too, you'll need those calories!

During lactation you'll need more protein than the adult male—at least seventy-five grams. This is because much of the protein you take in is secreted in the milk you give your child. Drinking six glasses of milk (preferably, nonfat fortified milk) in conjunction with a well-balanced diet daily should take care of these needs. Since your baby depends on your milk for all his needs, your diet should be planned to ensure that your milk supply is optimal.

If you are breast-feeding your infant, you will want to follow this general diet plan:

milk: (low fat or skim), minimum of three to four glasses, frequently five to six glasses.
vegetables and fruits: four ounces of orange juice or other citrus product, one serving of dark-green leafy or yellow vegetables, two additional servings of fruits and vegetables.
bread and cereal: at least four slices of bread or servings of cereal.

And you should drink a great deal of liquid. The actual quantity of milk produced is variable, but it can be close to a quart a day. Since human milk is about 90 percent water, you need to replace what is secreted. Failure to do so could impair the kidneys.

When you are planning your own diet, you are at the same time planning that of the baby that is depending on you. Practically all compounds that enter your body will be secreted in varying forms in the milk. You should, then, give careful consideration to drug and alcohol intake, and should eliminate cigarettes as nicotine, in addition to decreasing milk volume, may be harmful to the infant.

YOUR DIET AND THE PILL

There have been few drugs which have been as widely prescribed, enthusiastically praised, bitterly condemned, the subject of heated discussion in both medical and lay circles, as the oral contraceptive.

The current estimate is that some 10 million American women are now using The Pill—and millions of others have tried and discontinued it. There are a variety of types of oral contraceptives, the so-called "sequentials" which offer a synthetic form of estrogen for the first portion of the menstrual cycle and a combination of estrogens and progesterone in the latter part—and the "combination" type pills, which contain estrogen and progesterone in all tablets. In addition, there is a choice of dose levels and brands. But all together, the drugs fit the general category "The Pill."

Knowledge about the physiological effects of the oral contraceptive is still accumulating. Our knowledge about Pill safety and side effects was greatly clarified recently with the release of an international series of medical reports confirming a deadly, synergistic relationship of Pill use and cigarette smoking. Women who smoke moderately or heavily *and* use the oral contraceptive run significently higher risks of heart disease (myocardial infarction) than do nonsmoking Pill users. This was both bad news (for those who smoke) and good news for nonsmokers in that the report said that in effect, The Pill is much safer than previously thought since much of the sickness attributed to its use can really be explained by its use in conjunction with cigarettes.

The general side effects of The Pill have received a great deal of attention. But what hasn't been discussed very often in the popular press is the effect The Pill has on nutritional status and on body metabolism in general. Given that over fifty metabolic changes occur when you are "on The Pill"—including effects on dietary fats, carbohydrate, protein, mineral and vitamin metabolism—the topic is worth some serious attention.

Because hormone levels among Pill users are elevated (due to the fact that they are taking daily tablets with synthetic hormones) it is tempting to say the metabolic and nutritional changes of Pill

use is like being "a little bit pregnant." In some senses this is true
in that there is fluid retention, breast enlargement and weight gain
in both circumstances (in pregnancy, the weight gain, not counting
that attributable to the growing fetus, is about ten pounds, in Pill
use usually around six pounds). But the analogy doesn't hold up
very much longer than that. There are some "nutritional pluses and
minuses" associated with Pill use—not all of them parallel the
metabolic events and needs of the pregnant woman.

The Pluses

If you take The Pill, your body will need less of certain minerals—
and at least one vitamin.

Your iron needs, for instance, will be decreased. This is of particular interest in that iron deficiency is the most widespread nutritional problem in women and unlike the circumstances of oral
contraceptive use, the iron deficiency is aggravated by pregnancy
since not only does the growing fetus demand a great deal of it, but
a significant amount of blood—and thus iron reserves—is usually lost
during childbirth. When you are taking The Pill, however, there is
no growing fetus and, in addition, there is considerably less blood
loss during each menstrual period, as compared to the bleeding in
non-Pill related cycles.

Further, unlike pregnancy, Pill use does not appear to drain
calcium supplies. Indeed, The Pill seems to increase the intestinal
absorption of calcium and decrease its removal from bones. The
presence of estrogen in the oral contraceptive also is associated with
marked increases in the serum level of copper, a trace mineral
necessary for the formation of hemoglobin, the oxygen-carrying
component of blood.

A plus that could possibly be a minus is vitamin A, a nutrient
whose levels are increased with Pill use (and during pregnancy)
due to the effects of higher levels of estrogen. Excessive levels of
vitamin A can be toxic and particularly damaging to the liver, the
organ which stores vitamin A. So a woman on oral contraceptive
therapy should not be taking high dose supplements of this vitamin.

The Minuses

Vitamin B$_6$

Vitamin B$_6$, the inclusive name for pyridoxine, pyridoxal and pyridoxamine, plays an important role in protein metabolism, especially in the conversion of the amino acid tryptophan to the vitamin niacin. There is evidence that Pill users (and pregnant women) often experience some deficiency in this vitamin, although it is usually only a slight one. True deficiencies which occur infrequently in this country are characterized by hyperirritability, convulsions and anemia.

There have been a number of suggestions in the medical literature that slightly lower than normal levels of vitamin B_6 (and possibly some other nutrients as well) account, at least in part, for the occurrence of symptoms of depression, tiredness, lethargy, sadness or loss of libido which are reported in some 10-50 percent of oral contraceptive users. The explanation here is that there is some impairment of the metabolism in the brain of tryptophan, an essential amino acid, causing these behavioral changes. But there have been few studies made of this subject, and since depression can be induced by so many factors, it is difficult to attribute it exclusively to a dietary cause. Thus, the relationship of depression and vitamin B_6 deficiencies as they may occur during oral contraceptive therapy remains a speculative one.

You can get vitamin B_6 from a variety of sources: meats are particularly high in this nutrient, but other good sources include whole grains, bananas, lima beans, cabbage, potatoes, spinach, liver and kidney, and milk and milk products.

Folacin

Folacin, another B vitamin (also known as folate or folic acid), plays a vital role in the formation of nucleic acids, and this is necessary for all cell growth and production, functioning also in the degradation of amino acids. A number of studies have indicated that women on The Pill have lower than average serum levels of folacin (although not all of them do). When it occurs, it appears to be the result of The Pill's hormones impairing absorption of this nutrient or increasing the rate of removal of folacin from blood plasma.

Again, although Pill users could probably benefit from eating more foods which contain folacin, there is little reason to believe that a serious deficiency will develop if you are eating anything that approaches a balanced diet. Folacin deficiencies generally occur only in conjunction with other health problems—sickle cell anemia, alcoholism, leukemia, pellagra. When it does occur, the symptoms include lesions of the alimentary canal and diarrhea, the latter condition leading to further depletion of the body supply of folacin.

About 20 percent of oral contraceptive users tested have enlarged cervical and vaginal cells, which is an early sign of slight folacin deficiency. But probably the greatest risk which goes with low body levels of folacin relates to pregnancy: during early pregnancy significant amounts of this nutrient are critical, and it is possible that a woman who is on The Pill for a number of years and then becomes pregnant immediately after discontinuing it, might not be fully nutritionally prepared for a healthy pregnancy.

Where do you find a good supply of folacin? Spinach and other green leafy vegetables are good sources, as are mushrooms, liver, kidney and various fruits and vegetables. There are smaller amounts in meats and cereals. An important factor to remember in planning a diet rich in folacin is that the amount present in the food served may be highly variable, depending on the preparation procedures you use. If carelessly prepared, foods can lose up to 90 percent of their folacin levels. Avoid storing fresh produce for more than a few days and cook these foods for the shortest possible amount of time.

B_{12}

Vitamin B_{12} (also known as cobalamin or cyanocobalamin) is needed to ensure the health of all body cells, but is particularly important to the nervous system, bone marrow and digestive tract.

About half of Pill users have lower than average levels of B_{12} in their systems (although the actual tissue levels of this vitamin appear not to be affected). Again, true deficiencies are rare, but when it does occur, pernicious anemia (so named because until recently it was invariably fatal) develops. The red blood cells become significantly larger, symptoms such as fatigue, glossitis (smoothness of the tongue), sore and cracked lips, and increased amount of hydrochloric acid in the stomach become evident.

Foods of animal origin contain varying but generally significant amounts of Vitamin B_{12}, plant products containing none. So unless you are a strict vegetarian, you should have no problem getting enough of this nutrient. If you do, for whatever reason, decide not to eat meat, then choose from a variety of animal products such as eggs, milk and cheese. These will meet your needs for B_{12}.

What to Eat While You're on The Pill

The nutritional and general metabolic implications of oral contraceptive use are just now being understood. In addition to the decreased needs of a Pill user for iron, calcium, copper and vitamin A, and her increased need for vitamin B_6, B_{12} and folacin, there may in the future be other nutrients which are shown to need adjustment on oral contraceptive therapy. For example, there is now some limited evidence that estrogen increases the rate of ascorbic acid breakdown, thus increasing the dietary need for vitamin C. And it has been known for a number of years that estrogen stimulates the blood levels of triglycerides, that is, fatty acids (but does not have any consistent effect on the body's cholesterol levels). The significance, if any, of this increase in triglycerides is not known.

In the meantime, the most practical advice for the woman on The Pill is to eat, in moderation, a variety of foods, making sure that you get a bit more of those foods which are rich in B_6, B_{12} and folacin. More and more physicians are now acknowledging that dietary assessment and nutritional counselling are an essential component of family planning and of keeping attuned to the possibility that some specific and minor deficiencies might develop.

Do you need vitamin or mineral supplements to compensate for some of the nutritional effects of the oral contraceptive? The *Journal of the American Dietetic Association* recently supplied an interim answer to this question: "Until further information is available, no definitive recommendation regarding use of nutritional supplements can be made." Until one is made, you'd be best off not buying supplements, unless recommended by your physician, and spending your money in the grocery store on enjoyable, nourishing meals.

BABIES: THEY NEED GOOD NUTRITION TOO!!

What is a baby? A baby is not just any small animal, but a human infant—yours and mine. A baby is not a small edition of an adult. He is, in fact, a quite different organism. Though volumes have been written about the art and practice of child rearing, there are still great gaps in our knowledge. Let us consider some of the things we do know about the nutritional needs of babies.

We would like to emphasize that for infants, even more than for adults, nutrition cannot be separated from care—a baby must be "nurtured as well as nourished."

A newborn infant needs two to three times as many calories per pound of body weight as an adult. We may need only about twenty to thirty Calories a pound, but the baby will require forty-five to fifty Calories. When he is three or four weeks old, especially if he is large and active, he may be really hungry and need as much as fifty to sixty Calories per pound. After about six months a baby's growth rate slows down a little so that by the time he is a year old he may again need about forty-five to fifty Calories per pound.

These calories are best supplied by milk, which has approximately twenty Calories per ounce (mother's and cow's).

Thus, about 2½ ounces of milk per pound of baby will meet the energy needs for growth and activity. In fact, milk will meet most of a baby's nutritional needs for the first six months of life, except for iron, vitamin D, and vitamin C. You should generally feed small babies about once every three hours, every four hours for a larger one. Gradually you'll find you can omit that middle of the night feeding.

Human milk is the food most suited to the nutritional needs of the human infant. It has a good ratio of calories from proteins, carbohydrates, and fats. It is relatively foolproof as far as safety and sanitation are concerned.

Cow's milk in a variety of forms has been scientifically modified to make bottle-feeding as satisfactory physiologically as breast-milk feeding, though authorities stress the emotional importance of breast-feeding to both mother and child. Both human and cow's milk are good sources of most minerals and vitamins, except for iron and vitamin C in the case of cow's milk. A great variety of commercially made infant feeding formulas are also available about which your physician can advise you. But breast-feeding for the first few months is still the best for baby and mother.

Many new mothers find themselves in a quandary about whether or not to breast-feed. Inevitably they are surrounded by many sources of unsolicited and conflicting advice. In some cases practical considerations—a mother's need to return to work, for instance—might settle the question. But more often the question is more complex.

Basically, the decision of breast versus bottle feeding is a matter of personal preference. Psychological—and physical—factors and family relationships may enter the decision. For one woman, breast-feeding may be an excellent way to establish a close, emotional maternal tie with her child, offering an opportunity for expression of love and warmth. For another woman, these same feelings and mother-child bonding can develop without breast-feeding. Still other women may find it physically difficult or impossible to breast-feed, a situation which often makes her feel—unnecessarily—inadequate. In making this decision, remember that there is no one "right way." Individual circumstances determine what is "right."

There is no question that human milk is ideal for most infants, but cow's milk does have its advantages. Consider this comparison:

> Cow's milk contains more than three times as much protein as human milk.
> Human milk is twice as high in carbohydrate as cow's milk.
> Calcium levels are approximately four times higher, phosphorus about six times higher in cow's milk.
> Cow's milk is about four times higher in riboflavin than human milk.

Yet we do know that infants on cow's milk grow somewhat more slowly in the first few months, then a bit later begin to grow more quickly than those being breast-fed. This seems contradictory, but it isn't. Although cow's milk has more protein, the nature of that protein is such that it is not as easily digested in the first weeks of life by the infant as is the protein in breast milk. But scientifically prepared formula can reduce or eliminate these probems and, for all practical purposes, make human and cow's milk nutritionally comparable.

In making your decision on this subject, take your personal preferences into account along with your doctor's advice. Whichever decision you make—breast-feeding, or bottle-feeding with specially prepared formula, ideally designed to the needs of the infant—you can be sure your baby is going to be well-fed.

If the mother is well-nourished there is little need for supplementation of any kind before three months of age. A healthy baby is born with at least a three-month supply of iron, copper, and vitamin A stored in his liver. Some supplementary sources of vitamin C and

D are commonly recommended after the first months of life. Evaporated or fluid milk fortified with vitamin D provides the latter, as does most any kind of infant vitamin preparation. The vitamin supplement should also provide vitamin C, or this can come from a few swallows of orange juice. The newer vitamin preparations also have a small amount of the mineral nutrient fluoride, which is necessary for building teeth with maximum resistance to decay. A vitamin preparation with fluoride is particularly important to use if you live in a community that is still "backward" and has not yet fluoridated its water.

At about three months, it is advisable to provide additional sources of iron in the form of solid or semi-solid food. Cereals with iron added are preferred.

You should be careful of not overdoing the first solid foods. To you, a can or jar of baby food looks small. But to an infant it is an overwhelming feast. Give the child about half a teaspoon in the first day and just a bit more after that. Don't keep the can or jar around more than three or four days after you've opened it, even if it means you have to throw some out.

A recent study of infants in the Boston area showed that it is common practice to give babies more protein and a much higher calorie intake than is recommended by the National Research Council. This really represents "overfeeding." It is important to emphasize the fact that equating size with health is a questionable practice. Bigger babies are not necessarily better babies. In fact, there is a growing feeling in the fields of pediatrics and nutrition that fatness in your baby is no more desirable than in you. A fat baby often becomes a fat child or a child who is a feeding problem. We know now that adult weight-control problems often have their roots in poor infant-feeding practices.

Even for very young infants, eating time is more than just a biologically-determined occasion. A baby spends so much time sleeping, his meal times represent his main contact with the world. He needs more than nutrients at this time—he needs love, patience and a pleasant environment. Feeding a baby can prove a bit trying at times.

As your baby gets older, say seven to nine months old, you can make the transition from pureed to adult food. Baby-food manufacturers have what they call "junior foods" which are fairly finely chopped, but are different in texture from the pureed variety. By then the child likely will be on a three-meals-a-day schedule with midmorning and midafternoon snacks.

Your infant or young child does not need any of those protein supplement products often on sale in so-called health-food stores. Neither do elderly persons, and those with chronic or acute liver or kidney diseases may actually harm themselves. Contrary to what some merchants may tell you, no typical American of any age needs protein supplements.

The ingestion of excessive amounts of protein by infants creates health hazards, a well-documented medical fact. Infants in this country presently consume, on the average, two to four times as much protein as they need. Indeed, protein consumption is now so high that many infants are near the threshold of danger, and supplements can create substantial health risks.

Excessive protein can lead to a state of dehydration in a matter of hours and can overburden the infant's digestive and excretory system, causing kidney failure, coma and even death. The health problems from too much protein for children age one to three are also substantial, although not as great as for infants.

Protein supplements may be dangerous also for those with liver or kidney ailments because of the inability of those damaged organs to handle the demands produced by the metabolism of high levels of protein.

Not only are these supplements potentially hazardous but they are a very expensive source of protein. According to a recent Federal Trade Commission survey, the cost of ten grams of usable protein from protein supplements is about four times the cost of the protein in ordinary food such as bread, eggs, milk, cheese, peanut butter, chicken, fish, hamburger and even sirloin steak. So skip the protein supplements and stick to a well-balanced diet. It will be considerably cheaper to eat—and it will taste much better, too.

Preschool-Age Children

When your child is about two years old, you'll notice a dramatic—and normal change—in eating habits. His appetite will be reduced significantly. But this should not be a concern to you! Because his body growth is slowing down—and he will in the future grow more gradually—he is in need of less food.

Feeding a preschool-age child may prove to be a challenge. He'll want to eat "normal" foods but may find that many meats are too tough for his limited chewing ability. He will undoubtedly need some help. A satisfactory serving for a preschooler may be as small as only one tablespoon of meat for each age, so don't push the food. Your child may well be "finicky" about certain foods, particularly new vegetables, or may just go on "food jags" where he insists upon just one menu. Bear with it, and he will outgrow these. Particularly if he sees other members of the family enjoying food he rejected, he'll gradually change his attitude. You should try to have your child accept dark-green and yellow vegetables such as broccoli, kale, carrots and sweet potatoes to ensure he is getting enough vitamin A, a problem for some children today in this country.

Here are some specific tips on feeding a preschool-age child: Stick to a schedule for meals. For you a half-hour delay in dinner may be fine, but to a hungry child it could seem like an eternity. Generally serve foods with mild flavors and aromas. Young children are very sensitive and have a large number of functioning tastebuds. The same thing goes for extreme temperatures—avoid them because they are not well received by a child with a mouth more sensitive than ours.

Again, avoid foods which are difficult to chew. Always beware of any food which presents the possibility of causing a choking hazard. And serve children small-sized portions, telling them to come back for seconds. Some children get fat because they are told to "eat everything on their plate." Finally, don't bribe children into eating their dinner; that's not the way to teach good nutrition.

SCHOOL DAYS—AND THE FOURTH R—
Refueling With the School Lunch

Most parents make a real effort to supervise properly the feeding of their babies and little children. But the busy schoolchild is hard to catch—and watch. Here is the time we begin to run into trouble.

Each fall every school, large and small, is filled with peppy youngsters invigorated after a healthy summer. How long do they stay in this top physical condition? Do they remain handsomely strong or do they soon begin to droop?

Let's face it, much of the answer to that vital question is up to us—because innumerable children lag behind for just one simple reason: they aren't properly fed.

There's plenty of food in the United States. Yet still there are thousands and thousands of children in every part of the country, in every section of every city, who could do better if they ate the right foods.

Many children seem lazy when actually, having rushed off to school with little or no breakfast, they're just plain hungry. Others show the telltale marks of deficient nutrition: dull eyes, poor posture, fatigue, irritability, and listlessness. A multitude of unsatisfactory report cards can be blamed in part simply on poor food.

A car gives the best service when it has gas and oil and proper care. Likewise with children, top performance in classes and in sports requires an adequate supply of the nutrients necessary for growth and activity. Bright eyes, alert minds, well-coordinated muscles all depend on good nutrition. Schoolchildren need to learn good food habits as well as reading, writing and 'rithmetic.

This is a big challenge for mothers and fathers. Building better bodies and better students calls for planning by informed parents. In this instance, a little knowledge can produce enormous benefits.

The task isn't hard. What schoolchildren need is essentially what all the family needs. Only the quantities are different. Kindergarteners eat smaller portions than the older children; teen-agers need more than their parents.

Yet the principles are the same. Everyone at every age needs three meals a day, eaten without haste and in a pleasant atmosphere. Everyone at every age needs a variety of wholesome foods to supply proteins, minerals, vitamins, fiber and energy from carbohydrates and fats.

A good day begins with a good breakfast—fruit, milk, or cocoa made with milk; toast with margarine, and cereal with milk.

French toast or pancakes may occasionally be substituted for the cereal. Raisins may be added to the cereal for variety and minerals too. It's fine to combine but not to skimp. Breakfast should be a must for children and parents alike.

Lunch is equally important. A candy bar isn't a meal; a quick snack isn't necessarily a good lunch. The noon meal has to furnish food needs for a whole afternoon's duties, so it can't be slighted. The pattern is easy and flexible: some protein, such as cheese or a slice of meat; bread; a glass of milk; vegetable (as carrot, celery or tomato); and a serving of fruit. Candy, cookies, or ice cream come last—to top off the meal, not to substitute for it!

Then, if dinner includes a serving of meat, chicken or fish, a potato, a vegetable, and milk, the schoolchild will be well-fed. Sweets are fine, but again, at dessert time!

This is the design for eating that promotes fitness for school and for living, with, of course, the adults setting a good example.

Lunch Away from Home

By definition, school-age children are not always at home at mealtime. Many of them eat at school, either by taking a packed lunch or by eating a meal prepared in the school cafeteria. These school lunch programs are important, and it's worthwhile to spend a page or two in discussing them.

The majority—but not all—of the schools in this country have school lunch programs. The pity of this is that many of the schools which do not have them are the very ones in which the children need them most.

The usual lunch provided through the National School Lunch Program, the "Type A" lunch, follows a pattern set by our Department of Agriculture and is planned to provide approximately one-third of the daily nutritional requirements of a student of ten to twelve years of age.

The "Type A" lunch pattern is as follows:

1) Two ounces cooked lean meat, poultry or fish; or two ounces of cheese, one egg, or one-half cup cooked dried beans or dried peas; or four tablespoons of peanut butter; or an equivalent quantity of a combination of two of these items, served as a main dish, and one other menu item.

2) Three-quarters of a cup of two or more vegetables or fruit, or both. Green leafy or yellow vegetables and vitamin C-rich fruits are stressed.

3) One slice of whole-grain or enriched bread or the equivalent.

4) One-half pint of fluid milk; flavored or unflavored, whole, low-fat or skim milk or cultured buttermilk.

That's quite a meal, isn't it? And one of the best nutritional buys you'll ever come across, since the program is heavily supported by the contributions of the federal government. But can you imagine eating all of it in ten or fifteen minutes? No? Well, there are many schools in which the lunch lines are so long and the lunch periods so short that by the time the students get through the line, get their trays to the table, and start to eat, they're supposed to be back in class. Ten or fifteen minutes is too short a time to eat a meal the size of a school lunch without getting indigestion, and in many schools it results in some of the nutritious food left on the trays unconsumed.

If you find from questioning your child that this is the case in your school, then why not take action either through the P. T. A. or other groups connected with the school to try to remedy the situation. Schools run under tight schedules, and it's a tremendously difficult problem to feed a large number of children in a short time, especially when cafeterias are often not set up as well as they could be due to lack of funds or to antiquated equipment. The great problem here isn't the school personnel, who usually have the best intentions, but simply old Father Time. Nevertheless, if it exists in your child's school, examination and discussion of the problem with school personnel can result in a plan for effective action. More children should be encouraged to use the facilities. At the same time, the facilities and the lunchroom environment should be improved if necessary so that more children can be handled faster and the time that the students have to do the eating lengthened. But remember, very little can be done by simply registering complaints; mutual responsibility is the only answer. The school lunch program is an extremely useful part of the efforts in this country for nutritional betterment of our schoolchildren and is now in its third decade. Let's all make an effort to see that it is used to its fullest. Children who eat the lunch can receive lifelong health benefits from it.

You noticed that milk is included in all standard lunches. But some children prefer flavored milk or because of a special diet require nonfat milk.

So why no chocolate or skimmed milk? The answer we got from several authorities was cost. Chocolate milks, they said, cost more. And states have varying rules about the subsidy of chocolate milk; some allow reimbursement for it, but some do not. However, many children will not drink plain milk, so why not offer them a chocolate variety?

Originally there was no skimmed milk or the popular "2% milk" permitted in the school lunch program. Fortunately, these regulations have been changed to allow children to select these lower fat milks rather than whole, if they prefer. Both obesity and heart disease are major problems in our country. Skimmed milk, having fewer calories, should help the many children and teenagers for whom obesity is a major problem. And since there is substantial evidence that dietary changes—such as less saturated fat and cholesterol and more polyunsaturated fat—can help prevent or delay heart disease, it is good that children be allowed skimmed and low-fat milk if they wish it.

Steps should be taken to urge changes in existing school lunch programs so that state and local rules are not more restrictive than federal regulations, especially when these changes can make a positive contribution to our children's health. Why not make it part of your business to see that one of the real nutritional bargains offered by your government is used to its fullest advantage?

But back to the general topic.

Not all schools who have a lunch program participate in the National School Lunch Program. Those schools who do not may not follow a sound nutritional meal pattern or may allow students to select any food they wish. In our opinion, the National School Lunch Program is good and should continue to be an integral part of our educational system. While its initial aim is to see to it that children have at least one nutritious meal a day, the children, the teachers, the parents, and ultimately our civilization reap some very important auxiliary benefits.

A child who is fed properly is a better student than a hungry one. A couple of years ago, we did a little study of nutritional status in two Boston area elementary schools. While over 25 percent of the children had no or unsatisfactory breakfasts, over one-third of them had very poor lunches. These schools had no school lunch program. The children brought their lunches or bought them on the way to school. You can imagine what a ten-year-old with thirty-five cents for lunch would buy! The lunches were eaten in the classrooms. There was little attempt on the part of the teachers to pay attention to what the children were eating. Some of the teachers were unaware that some children had no lunch day after day. In fact, some teachers even made a little fun of the school nurse's attempts to talk about proper meals. We were impressed by the short attention spans, by the restlessness, the apathy of many of the students. We are convinced that if these children had had the benefit of a proper meal many problems would have been solved.

About 85 percent of the total U.S. school population is in schools which participate in the National School Lunch Programs. This should be 100 percent. And, only half the children in participating schools take advantage of the lunch program. This is unfortunate. Believe it or not, only part of the "hungry child" problem is economic. Children from middle- and high-income groups are frequently poorly nourished—because of lack of supervision, ignorance or indifference.

Why not make it part of your business to see that one of the real nutritional bargains offered by your government is used to its fullest advantage? Support your National School Lunch Program!

THOSE PERILOUS TEEN YEARS

There are a number of good reasons for concern about the food habits of teen-agers.

First, nutritional demands in this period are at their maximum. The growth spurt preceding sexual maturation generally occurs in girls between ages eleven and thirteen, in boys between ages thirteen and fifteen. Bodies grow rapidly then. Indeed, in the ages fourteen to sixteen a girl's body requires more nutrients than at any other time in her life, with the exception of pregnancy and lactation. For a boy the peak nutritional demands occur around ages fourteen to eighteen.

Second, adolescents are generally casting off their habits of childhood and trying to establish their own identities. Part of this struggle may be the rejection of the diet advice they have been getting at home. As a result, too often teen-agers are careless, skipping breakfast, going on fad diets and filling up on snack foods, which by themselves do not provide good nutrition. This time of transition is also a period of emotional upheaval, a condition which often makes healthy eating difficult, although not impossible.

Third, teen-agers are well-known for their susceptibility to fads— including fad diets. As we'll discuss below, some of these food fascinations can pose serious health problems.

Fourth, the habits formed as a teen-ager lay the groundwork for his entire adulthood eating pattern. It is important that from the beginning, his expression of individuality in the diet department emphasize nutritious, well-balanced meals.

It's never too early to think about good nutrition habits. We know, for instance, that our thousands of annual heart attack victims do not succumb because of what they ate in their fifties and sixties. Their susceptibility to this disease started many, many years before, and we feel that diet may have a great deal to do with that susceptibility. Some years ago, doctors performing autopsies on young American soldiers were startled to discover that many of them already had signs of atherosclerosis in their coronary arteries. The average age was twenty-two. The beginnings of this atherosclerosis probably began early in adolescence, or even earlier.

What are good health eating habits, both in the teen years and later? Skim milk, more veal, fish and chicken, and less beef. Far fewer eggs, polyunsaturated margarines instead of butter—and, above all, smaller portions.

First, we must not forget that one out of every four mothers has her first child when she is less than twenty years old. So for a significiant minority of teenage girls, the nutrition requirements involve more than just one person.

"Do as I say, not as I do" won't work when it comes to good food habits. Teen-agers cannot do it alone. They need help, and this requires understanding and cooperation of parents and teachers.

When teen-agers are concerned about being fat or skinny, weak or weary, it is up to the adults to be available for advice. It is up to the leaders to set good examples and to practice what they preach.

Too often mother sets the pattern, and daughter follows suit, in the no-breakfast routine. For the rest of the day they cut down on meat, avoid bread, and the vegetables and fruits are few. What happens? They end up anemic.

Thousands and thousands of high-school girls all over the land do not get enough iron. They lack zip. They are not alert for classes and dates. Iron-rich foods just cannot be bypassed.

Boys skimp on lunch. Then at dinner, like so many fathers, they go light on fruits and vegetables but heavy on pie and cake. Is that the kind of menu served at a training table? No! Athletes know that food makes a difference.

Watch the corner drugstore near the high school from eight to nine in the morning. It is mobbed with youngsters grabbing a quick "breakfast" before classes—quick and consisting of soda pop and a candy bar.

Calories are there, but a dearth of health-building nutrients. If they want to be fit, adults as well as children must base their meals on the Basic Four. No one can consistently cut nutritional corners and come out on top.

Parents of teens and even pre-teens must see that their boys and girls are receiving a well-balanced diet before they reach the stage of the capricious appetite, the "herd" influence, the fascination with the bizarre. A youngster who has had sound training in good food habits does not persist in bad ones too long.

Furthermore, healthful, attractive meals can and should be served at home at regular times. The whole family should be expected to be there and to eat everything.

Good food habits must be a joint project for mothers and fathers and teen-agers together. Are you parents helping your teen-agers to eat properly for strength now and health in the future? Are you setting good examples?

Some More Thoughts For Teen-agers

All teen-agers want to be healthy and happy. Boys and girls share the same ambition: to be attractive and well-liked. They all hope for clear skin, bright eyes, shiny hair. They all need the firm muscles and good posture that are basic to the best possible appearance. They all want plenty of energy for their work and their play. But not all teen-agers are well-nourished. The general conclusion from studies in this age group is that young men are better nourished than young women, probably because they take in more calories and allow themselves a greater opportunity for variety. Teen-age girls are often very concerned about having a slim body to meet their ideal requirements for sexual attractiveness. But in the process, sometimes their nutrition suffers.

Teen diets are often found to be low in calcium, ascorbic acid, vitamin A and, particularly for the teen-age girl, iron. This latter deficiency for her may result in low hemoglobin in the blood and a constant feeling of being tired. Again, if it goes far enough, insufficient iron may result in anemia.

Boys, on the other hand, more often see themselves as underweight. They generally consume more milk, cereal and meat than women, thus explaining why they are generally better fed.

Every teen-ager needs to know that good food is the foundation for health and vigor and glowing good looks. For bounce and well-being today, and for parenthood in the future, food intake is of paramount importance.

But—our teen-agers are not eating right, particularly our teen-age girls. What do these youngsters do?

1. They eat too many calories, or too few.

2. They shortchange themselves on protein, calcium, iron, vitamin A, ascorbic acid, thiamine, and riboflavin. As we mentioned above, girls are worse than boys in this respect, particularly concerning iron.

3. They have highly irregular eating habits and are inclined to go on binges. When criticized, they comment, "So what? As we grow older, we will settle down; all this is temporary."

Perhaps this is true and today's food habits are but temporary. But if and when they change, it may be too late. The damage will be done and it cannot be undone.

What damage?

The age period from thirteen to twenty years is the most critical one after the first three years of life. This is the time when size and shape are shifting from childhood's characteristics to adult dimensions. All the requirements for this accelerated growth must come from food.

Beware of Adolescent Food Faddism!

A faddist approach to nutrition is bad at any age, but in the adolescent years it can mean very serious trouble.

Researchers at the Nutrition Division in the Department of Community Medicine at the Mount Sinai School of Medicine have expressed concern about what they see to be a growing group of teen-agers who are adopting eccentric eating patterns, some of which are grossly restrictive. Again, faddism for a teen-ager is a way of establishing his independence, proving he or she is "different."

Vegetarianism—which we'll discuss in detail a few pages from now—may be particularly attractive to the adolescent who wants to "live simply, return to nature." You *can* eat well on a vegetarian diet—if you include milk and eggs—but most young adults do not approach vegetarianism scientifically. Occasionally, for instance, a wave of "fruitarians" whose mainstay is raw or dried fruits and nuts affects many of our country's youth. This is hardly a diet that will supply the nutrients of the Basic Four Food Groups. Nutritionally, it is fruitless!

Teen-agers frequently turn to fad diets for a few days and then return eagerly to normal eating patterns. But others have been known to approach food faddism, for instance, the infamous macrobiotic diet, with religious zealotry. In an earlier chapter we mentioned the young woman who starved to death on a rigorous diet of brown rice in an effort to reach the ultimate phase of enlightenment on the spiritual ladder. Evidence at the inquest into her death indicated that similar fatalities had occurred previously. These grim examples remind us of our responsibility in deterring teen-agers from bizarre eating sprees.

Well, What Should Teen-agers Eat?

See that you provide a well-balanced diet made up of a variety of foods chosen from the Basic Four. The teen-ager needs lots of foods, but not just calories. The recommended allowances for protein, calcium, and iron, as well as for calories, are considerably higher for the young adolescent than for an adult.

Here is a suggested menu that will provide all the essential nutrients in the proper amounts, except for calories. A sixteen-year-old girl probably needs about 2400 Calories a day. This menu supplies only 2000. So if the young miss really needs to trim down a bit, this will do it—at the rate of about two-thirds of a pound a week.

The idea is to see that three substantial meals of well-planned and attractive foods are provided and include a minimum of "snacks," unless they are something saved from a meal—such as fruit, milk, or a portion of a sandwich.

Breakfast	*Amount*	*Approximate Calories*
Orange or grapefruit or citrus juice or fresh fruit, such as melons or strawberries	1 medium serving	70
Cereal	½ cup	110
Toast with margarine	1 slice	110
Milk, whole	1 cup	165

Lunch	Amount	Approximate Calories
Sandwich with a generous serving from the meat group—e.g., hamburger (2 ounces) on bun or tuna-salad sandwich or peanut-butter sandwich	1	300
Celery and carrot sticks	1 serving	15
Apple (or other fruit)	1 medium	70
Milk, whole	1 cup	165

Dinner

Roast beef, meat loaf or chops (liver at least once a week)	3-ounce serving	300
Potato—baked or mashed or scalloped with	small serving	100
margarine	1 pat	50
Broccoli, or other dark green vegetable	½ cup	20
Lettuce salad with lemon or vinegar	1 serving	15
Jello with fruit	1 serving	100

Between-Meal Snacks

After school: Coke	1 glass	80
Bedtime: Milk, cookie	1 glass, 1 medium	265

Total Calories for the day, approximately   2,000

Again, if your teen-ager's weight does have to be reduced, make sure that he or she—most likely it will be "she"—does it wisely, avoiding the bizarre diets which regularly appear in women's magazines. The overweight teen-ager may be eating the same kinds of foods as his average friend, but too much of them. Also, most likely he or she is not getting enough exercise.

While we are speaking of teen-age diets, we should mention the problem of anorexia nervosa, a condition which sometimes develops particularly among young girls who take their dieting too seriously. If your dieting teen-ager loses the desired amount of weight, but continues to restrict calories severely to the point where he or she is markedly underweight, anorexia nervosa, a form of mental disturbance, may be the problem. Medical help there is a must.

NUTRITION IN THE GOLDEN YEARS

How and what should older people eat? This question is becoming of increasing importance to all of us. Life expectancy has increased considerably, and our population of older citizens is becoming larger all the time. In 1900 there were about 3 million people sixty-five years or older. By 1950 the figure was 12 million, and the 1970 census showed that we had over 20 million senior citizens. In the late 1970s, because of our unique demographic patterns, persons over age sixty-five will make up a very significant portion of the total population.

Our added years should be ones of enjoyment and pleasure. For this, our health is a must. Good health is dependent on good nutrition.

Of course, poor eating habits in early life as well as in later years influence health, but there are some points about nutrition for older people that we should keep in mind.

Aging and Calories

As one grows older, his amount of activity usually lessens. In fact, for most of us this restriction of activity begins about age twenty-five, when we start settling down to family and job. There is evidence that after age twenty-five the actual calorie requirement is reduced by about 5 percent for each decade. Thus, if at age twenty-five one maintained a steady weight on an intake of 3000 Calories per day, by age fifty-five this would be reduced by 15 percent, or to about 2550 Calories.

Older folks who have restricted activity need still fewer calories. Calories can be reduced by having smaller servings of the usual menus. Variety in food consumption remains important. The nutrition of older folks is frequently complicated by lack of funds to purchase enough food, poor teeth with which to chew (a good reason for fluoridation), and lack of interest in obtaining good nutrition. "Bachelors' scurvy" and "widows' anemia" are frequently due to boredom and lack of interest in obtaining a healthy diet. But so far as is now known, old age adds no unusual requirements for nutrients.

Surveys show that older people not only need fewer calories but, in fact, they actually eat less than younger adults. This means that more care in food selection must be exercised to be sure sufficient amounts of the essential nutrients are obtained within the limits of the decreased calorie needs.

As far as we now know, the needs for other nutrients such as protein, vitamins and minerals are not altered appreciably as people age. The older person adjusts much more slowly to stress and extremes than younger individuals. Extremes of temperatures, too much or too little food, too much or too little activity can all cause physiological and/or psychological upsets.

The concensus of opinion to date is that people over sixty-five should follow the same rules as younger ones in order to maintain health—using moderation as the keynote.

1. Avoid obesity or emaciation.
2. Select food with care from the "Basic Four" so it provides the essential nutrients and variety.
3. Eat frequent small meals rather than two or three large ones.
4. Indulge in moderate and regular activity but not so you become fatigued.

Although body needs for iron do not diminish with the years, the intake often drops. There are recent suggestions that iron intake is marginal. Meats are good sources of iron, but because meat can be costly, or difficult to prepare or to chew, it is often excluded by the elderly. It is advisable to stress the importance of a weekly serving of liver and of other iron-rich foods such as dried beans and peas, dark-green leafy vegetables, and whole-grain or enriched breads and cereals.

The role of fluoride and the value of supplemental fluoride in the treatment or prevention of osteoporosis in the elderly is important. An optimal intake of fluoride through the use of fluoridated water, is beneficial to the elderly as it is to everyone else.

With vitamins, as with minerals, needs of the elderly are unchanged, but intakes are often poor. When foods are not carefully chosen, the supply of vitamins is usually far from adequate, and vitamin C is often missing entirely. This may be due to a widespread tendency to classify fruit juices as "hard-to-digest," "acid" foods. Since fruits and juices, which supply ascorbic acid, are easily obtained, require no preparation and need not cause digestive difficulties, the desirability of reeducation is obvious. Deficiency of other vitamins, too is often a result of ignorance. The best way, even for the elderly, to obtain all of the vitamins, as well as all of the other essential nutrients, is through a variety of foods selected from the Basic Four Food Groups.

The goal for all adults is to maintain "desirable weight," which is the average weight according to sex and height at age twenty-five. To achieve this necessitates for many a gradual decrease in caloric intake, since with advancing years there is a progressive decrease in activity and hence in energy requirements.

Those individuals are fortunate who have kept their calories in balance and have maintained a desirable weight. All others should be advised to regulate calorie intake and output (physical activity) so that desirable weight is reached and maintained.

No survey of nutritional requirements is complete without mention of water. Inadequate intake of liquids is characteristic of the elderly and a common cause of constipation. Older people need to be reminded to have six to seven glasses of fluid per day.

Fiber is also indicated to prevent or treat constipation. Frequently, individuals do not realize the value of cooked fruits and vegetables in this connection. Whole-grain breads and bran cereals are good sources of fiber. Many adults need information to counter their queer notions about "roughage" and their preconceived, often stubborn, opinions about the desirability of avoiding certain fruits or vegetables or whole-grain products.

Will vitamin pills and special food preparations help? Usually not unless they are prescribed by a physician for a good reason.

Several studies have shown that half or more people buying vitamins were wasting their money because they already had good diets and didn't need supplements. Nearly three-quarters of the others were wasting their money also because they were purchasing preparations that failed to supply the particular vitamins lacking in their particular diets. All of these people would have been far wiser—and healthier—if they had relied on a good variety of foods which would provide *all* of the vitamins and also *all* of the other fifty or more nutrients needed.

Eating nutritiously in the golden years can present a real challenge to some people—particularly those who are living alone and on a fixed income. A higher probability of health problems make older people particularly vulnerable to the claims of "health food" merchants, and money that otherwise could be spent on a variety of nutritious foods is gambled on a worthless "potion" which suggests it can perform the functions of a fountain of youth.

Nutrition for the elderly is a topic which is drawing an increasing amount of attention—and in the next few years as the over sixty-five-age population expands, you're likely to hear even more about it. We, as a society, are at last accepting the responsibility of aiding our older citizens, many of whom are lonely and lacking the incentive to cook regular nutritious meals. The rapidly growing "meals on wheels" program is an example of the community interest in this area. Find out what similar programs your neighborhood offers, and support them!

VEGETARIANISM—AND ITS VARIETIES

One of the classic stories about vegetarianism was told by the novelist Leo Tolstoy. A Russian woman accepted an invitation to Tolstoy's home for dinner and found a live chicken tied to her chair. "My conscience forbids me to kill it," Tolstoy said. "As you are the only guest taking meat I would be greatly obliged if you would undertake the killing first."

For Tolstoy, and many individuals, there are religious reasons for not killing and eating animals. But today, there is a growing interest in vegetarianism which goes beyond religious doctrine. Political-ecological arguments, concerns about threatening the food chain, and complaints about "chemicals" in meat have led to the emergence of "new vegetarians" who claim, among other things, that it is not morally right in the time of a food crisis to eat meat—particularly red meat—especially when it takes seven or eight pounds of grain to produce one pound of beef.

Of course, the choice of a vegetarian lifestyle is an individual one. Here we are only interested in its nutritional aspects. Can you be healthy and a vegetarian at the same time?

The answer is "yes," but there are some qualifications. First, consider that there are varieties in vegetarians. A pure, strict vegetarian diet excludes all animal foods—meat, poultry, fish—and products of animal origin—eggs, milk, cheese, ice cream and related products. An extreme version of this would preclude acceptance of vaccinations because they are prepared from animal cultures.

Then there is what is known as a "lacto-vegetarian" which, while they exclude meats and fish, allow dairy products, but not eggs. A "lacto-ovo-vegetarian" permits eggs and dairy products, but no direct consumption of fish and meat.

If you are a strict vegetarian, it is difficult to stay healthy because such a diet will be low in some of the essential amino acids and devoid of vitamin B_{12}. Healthy vegetarian eating is easy if you consume milk, eggs and cheese. The following diet, for instance, would be as nutritious as a meat diet.

Breakfast: Fruit or fruit juice, cereal and milk or egg, toast and jam, glass of milk.

Mid-morning snack: Glass of milk or fruit juice.

Lunch: Glass of milk, cheese sandwich, fruit for dessert.

Afternoon snack: Glass of milk or fruit juice or a handful of nuts.

Dinner: Three vegetables, one of which should be peas or beans; an egg, bread, glass of milk, and fruits, nuts or cheese for dessert.

The only real problems arise when you omit the eggs, milk and milk products. You may recall from an earlier chapter that only animal products have the necessary nutrient, vitamin B_{12}. Examples of the deficiency of this vitamin are stunted growth in children, irritability and other indications of nerve malfunction. For strict vegetarians, supplements of vitamin B_{12} are a must.

MEAL PLANNING FOR SPECIAL DIETS

We could write a complete separate book on how to plan diets for different medical conditions. Just a discussion of food allergies alone could take up many pages. But here, instead, we'll just give you some brief comments on only two of the more common special diets.

Eating Without a Grain of Salt

Can it be done? No. Because salt is everywhere. But you can cut down on salt. That's a good idea for most of us, but for certain individuals, existing health conditions—for instance, high blood pressure—make it a must. They must turn to a low-sodium diet.

Salt and baking soda and the foods containing them are the main sources of sodium in the diet. Milk and its products also provide a generous amount of sodium.

If you need to lower your salt intake, there are a few simple things you can do. First of all, give your saltshakers away, both the ones on the table and those in your kitchen cabinets. Next, eat less of those foods in which additional salt is used in their preparation, for example, ham and potato chips. Read your labels—especially on frozen and other prepared foods. Depending on how low your diet is to be in sodium, you may have to restrict milk and its products or use a low-sodium milk preparation.

Lastly, be careful you are not getting substantial amounts of sodium in toothpaste or mouthwashes. Ask your dentist or pharmacist to recommend low sodium products.

Look in your supermarket and you'll see all types of salt-substitutes and low sodium products. Life in general and meals in particular can still be fun without saltshakers!

"My Cholesterol Level Is High!"

Ernest Holsendolph, writing in *The New York Times*, tells of the day he received a letter from Rockefeller University Hospital: "Recently you gave a pint of blood to the New York Blood Program," it began. "Nothing to worry about, but we'd just like to see you," the letter continued. He found the note about as reassuring as one from the Internal Revenue Service, and he quickly appeared at the hospital. "Too much cholesterol in your blood," he was told. "You have nothing to be concerned about unless you are interested in living a long time!"

Mr. Holsendolph then set out to lower his cholesterol. He was told to lose some weight and change his diet. "Butter, eggs, whole milk, those beautifully marbled steaks, cheeses—all those wonderful things were limited," he complained. In its place, no more than four ounces of trimmed red meat in a day (no more than twenty ounces a week) were permitted. Liver, sweetbreads and shellfish were also on the "watch out for" list. The rest of his diet was to be composed of low cholesterol dishes—fish, poultry, vegetables, fruits.

And a few weeks into the diet, he found it wasn't so bad after all. Margarines with a corn or safflower oil base, rich in polyunsaturated oils made potatoes—and popcorn—taste delicious. Specially made salad dressings prepared with polyunsaturated oils made excellent mouth-watering salads. Gourmet dishes could be easily made with veal and chicken. And Chinese restaurants with their use of lean meats and food fried in vegetable oil (normally without the prohibited coconut ingredients) made excellent substitutes for French restaurants with escargot cooked in butter (and plenty of it).

Mr. Holsendolph's diet worked. He soon dropped his cholesterol level from 296 to 218. And you can do it too. Being on a low cholesterol diet is not like switching from color television to black and white. Low cholesterol diets can be glamorous—and they need not mean that foods such as eggs or an occasional splurge with "forbidden foods" are never allowed. It just means making daily alterations which significantly reduce foods high in saturated fats, high in cholesterol and substitute those health-promoting fats high in unsaturates, particularly the polyunsaturates.

If you want some specifics on planning a diet to lower your blood cholesterol, see your doctor, write your Heart Association and follow the recipes we suggest (see Appendix). Here we'll settle for a summary of the general rules which make up a diet to lower blood cholesterol:

1. Limit your total caloric intake. Make sure your weight is where it should be to maximize your chances for good health.

2. Decrease by half or more your consumption of saturated fats. Choose lean meats, cut down significantly on most cheese and butter. Increase your use of chicken, veal and fish.

3. Restrict egg yolks to two to three a week. Try those new cholesterol-free egg substitutes.

4. Increase your use of polyunsaturated oils (margarine and vegetable salad oils). Stay away from animal fats and coconut oil as much as possible. Read your labels! If a product simply says it contains "vegetable oil," the chances are good it is coconut oil and should be avoided. Use those products where the vegetable oil is identified as corn, safflower, soy, cotton-seed or sunflower.

There is one dietary adjustment which most all of us need to give attention: calorie intake and expenditure. That is a subject that deserves a whole chapter.

Chapter Seven
The New-Fangled Old-Fashioned "You've-Got-To-Eat-Less-To-Lose-Weight" Diet — Try It!

THE WOES OF (EXCESS) ADIPOSE

Average Americans eat as though they were fattening themselves up for the market.

In 1923, Henry T. Finck coined the term "girth control." In his book, *Girth Control for Womanly Beauty, Manly Strength and a Long Life for Everyone*, he advised readers to have a "gorgeous time without gorging." And the phrase and the general concept of weight control has long been with us and is very much a topic of interest today. Recent public opinion polls have indicated that some 55 percent of women and 38 percent of men weigh more than they wish they did—and a significant portion of them are overweight to the point where they are threatening their health. Only a small portion of us have the opposite problem—underweight.

Why do so many of us have to wage an ongoing battle against excess pounds? It's simple. We eat more than we need. We consume tasty, but very caloric foods and we generally lead sedentary lives. Somehow there is time for three generous meals plus liberal snacking frequently accompanied by drinks loaded with calories, but little time for exercising off the calories we have swallowed. Former Surgeon General Jesse Steinfield has summarized the plight of our sedentary society: "The only exercise some people get is jumping to conclusions, sidestepping responsibilities and pushing their luck." We agree. From our observations, many obese Americans limit their exercise to pushing down the toaster and pouring alcoholic beverages over ice cubes.

Let's begin our discussion of weight problems with the less common end of the spectrum—underweight. If you don't have this problem, don't read the next section! You may be unduly tempted and you'll certainly be jealous.

Underweight

Being "painfully" thin may not only be "painful" as far as appearance is concerned, but it is a definite health hazard as well. Severe underweight (twenty or more pounds below desirable weight), since it usually occurs in young people, can favor the development of serious diseases such as tuberculosis and anemia.

Lack of physical endurance, easy fatigability, inability to concentrate, susceptibility to digestive disturbances and to infections are some of the milder problems of the underweight.

The treatment for this situation seems simple enough: Eat more! But, as anyone who is or has been underweight knows, it is as difficult (or more so) to eat more as it is to eat less. Careful planning and a thorough understanding of the factors involved are essential. A doctor's help is advisable.

There may be an organic disturbance responsible for the loss of weight or the inability to gain weight properly. However, in healthy people underweight is usually the result of poor living and eating habits. It requires effort and concentration to change these to more desirable ones.

There are a few suggestions we can offer that have been effective for others, and may help you:

1. *Plan* for three regular meals—at the same time each day if possible. The purpose here is to establish regular eating habits. Sit down at the table, whether you want to or not.

2. *Plan* to rest or relax for at least ten to fifteen minutes before each meal. Stop what you are doing, change your atmosphere—internal and external. This is to rest you physically and emotionally. Fatigue and tension are thieves of appetite.

3. *Plan* for some mild outdoor activity daily: walking (a dog is a fine help here), a little gardening—anything to improve the

circulation and stimulate your appetite. But don't overdo and wear yourself out.

4. *Think* about food! Read recipes, look at the lovely pictures of food in magazines and newspapers. Maybe go so far as to develop an interest in a certain type of cooking, such as becoming the barbecue expert of the neighborhood, or the Lasagna Queen.

5. *Eat frequently, but not within two hours before mealtime.* Eat a good breakfast, then half or three-quarters of an hour later eat a doughnut and milk, or drink a glass of eggnog. *Don't* eat foods at least two hours before regular meal hours, for this might dull your appetite. *Do* eat before you go to bed. Make this snack a fairly substantial one.

Try following these simple steps, and perhaps they will help you graduate from the "a rag, a bone, and a hank of hair" class. Just don't overdo it. Being a little underweight is usually better for you than being a little overweight.

How Much Is Too Much?

The humorist-writer Jean Kerr has explained that you know you are too heavy when, as you leave your seat on a bus or subway, two people immediately replace you.

But there are more scientific approaches to the definition. You can begin by rechecking Tables 2 and 3 back in chapter three. If you are of medium frame, a female five-feet-five inches in height (with shoes with two-inch heels), and are age twenty-five or over, your desirable weight range with ordinary clothing is 116 to 130 pounds. Remember, desirable weights don't change after age twenty-five. Overweight means you are some 10 to 20 percent over your desirable body weight. An excess of 20 percent places you in the obese column.

A different test of overweight has been suggested by Dr. Carl C. Seltzer and Dr. Jean Mayer, both former members of Harvard's nutrition department. This test involves a simple measurement of the fat under the skin of the upper arm—a pinch test, with the size of that pinch scientifically measured.

But generally, one does not need fancy methods to determine whether or not you are overweight. If you have excess fat, you know it. The question is not which definition you are going to use to describe yourself—the question is what you are going to do about it.

DON'T TAKE OBESITY LIGHTLY!

Obesity *is* a weighty problem.   The paintings of Raphael, Leonardo, Michelangelo, suggest that being "pleasingly plump" was considered "in."   Indeed through much of our world history, plumpness was symbolic of social status and affluence. It was a sign that you were in generally good health, free from the ravages of, for instance, tuberculosis.

But today, obesity is both physically and medically unattractive. It is in itself a serious problem, and what is more, it causes an increase in the frequency and seriousness of most other diseases, particularly diabetes.

Studies have shown that middle-age men who are 30 percent or more over their normal weight have twice the risk of a heart attack compared with middle-aged men of normal weight. And it is known that extra pounds increase the risk of developing high blood pressure two to three times. The same study mentioned above found the risk of heart disease four times higher in people with high blood pressure as compared with those whose blood pressure was normal. Obesity also means greater likelihood of elevated blood cholesterol, strokes, and diabetes and increased chances of problems during pregnancy. Obesity is one of the "risk factors" in heart disease that can be controlled. The task may be difficult, but it's a good health investment.

Other facts and other experts all agree that obesity is a hazard, particularly when it is accompanied by other illnesses as it usually is in those over forty years of age. Slimness is needed not only for style, but more so for survival.

And you may be risking more than your physical health by assuming the role of the Great Fatsby. Caesar may have wanted fat men about him, but the fact is that many employers don't.   It's simply a matter of appearance, and many people relate fatness with laziness or assume that obesity may be a sign of physical or psychological conditions which may interfere with work.

More recent studies suggest that college admission chances may be diminished among obese high school seniors. Overweight can be a social problem at most any point in life.

The popular 1947 song, "I don't want her, you can have her, she's too fat for me," brought a valid social message. While we do love Santa Claus despite his "little round belly that shook when he laughed like a bowl full of jelly," fat people generally have more trouble being accepted. They are generally unhappy with their own self-image and are frustrated that they never seem to look right in the clothes that look great in store windows. (It is said that more diets begin in dress shops than in doctors' offices). It is interesting to note that formerly fat people report increased self-confidence and pride in their appearance as well as being able to move around more freely.

So decide to be a loser. The benefits—both social and medical—are great.

"But I Hardly Eat Anything!"

Of course every individual is different. Not all overweight people are obese, nor are all overweight people, obese or not, in real danger because of their weight. Some look and feel better when they weigh somewhat more than their statistically desirable weight. However, if you are 20 percent above the upper range of your desirable weight you may be pretty sure that you are not in good shape, in any sense of the word, and you *are* obese. And the chances are that you are the way you are because you are eating and drinking too much of the wrong types of food and not burning up these extra calories in physical activity. Yes, we've got to face it, obesity is the result of the consumption of more calories than are burned up by the body. But there are many reasons for such apparent overeating. These are some of the more common causes:

1. Ignorance—both of the caloric values of foods and beverages, and also of the relationship of energy needs to energy intake and output.

2. Poor food habits—both in choice of foods and in eating patterns.

3. Faulty family patterns that result when parents indulge in meals that are top-heavy in calories and thus set disastrously bad examples for their children.

4. Failure to realize the need for cutting down on food intake as activity decreases.

5. Use of food as a comfort or diversion (instead of a book or a walk, a job or a hobby) to counteract feelings of worry or frustration or unhappiness.

6. The uncontrolled snack habit—which leads to uncounted, forgotten extras.

7. Genetic factors—which account for certain disturbances in fat metabolism in animals, and *may perhaps* apply in some cases to man.

This long list shows that we cannot summarize easily or quickly the cause and cure of overweight. Different causes explain different people's difficulties. We do know, though, that for nearly every individual obesity is risky business. It is wise to watch the scale, for an ounce of prevention is far easier and less painful than a pound of cure.

TIPS ON A LOSING PROPOSITION

Unless you are 20 percent or more over your desirable weight (in which case you should see a physician for advice) or in a hurry to lose those pounds which make you more than 10 percent over what you'd like to be, you needn't approach your meals with a paper, pencil and calorie counter. Just be sensible. Eat smaller portions, cut out frequent consumption of calorie-rich dishes, and always keep your eye on the Basic Four. Of course you should make sure you continue to get some physical activity and probably more than you are accustomed to.

But if you do feel the need to take off some pounds, and relatively quickly, consider our diet advice.

The first part of that advice is to avoid fad diets. We'll get into the specifics of the dieting nonsense which currently surrounds us a few pages from now, but here it is important to emphasize that gimmicks do not offer the road to quick and permanent weight loss. And neither do expensive arrays of "reducing equipment." All you need is willpower, determination, an awareness of the basics of nutrition and your own personal calorie needs, and two pieces of dietary apparatus—a scale and a mirror.

How to Lose Weight—and Like It

Are calories important? Do they count? Emphatically, yes! If you want your food and your weight to fit you and your needs you have to understand calories.

What, then, is a calorie?

As we discussed in chapter two, it is a measure of energy, just as a pound is a measure of weight. Breathing, moving, eating—everything the body does requires a certain number of calories of energy.

Where does the body obtain these calories? Chiefly from food. All foods, except pure and simple coffee, tea, and bouillon, contain calories, some more, some less. These are the source of body energy.

However, calories can also be obtained from stored body fat. On the other hand, if there are more food calories than can be burned, they are stored as excess body fat. The whole trick, then, is to keep the calories in balance.

If you eat more calories than your body requires, the extras are changed into fat. If you eat less than your body requires, the energy comes from stored fat. If you eat just what you need, you are in the clear, and in balance; you do not gain and you do not lose.

There are approximately 3,500 Calories in each stored pound of body fat. And the formula for shaking some of that fat is very simple: to reduce slowly, safely and surely, cut back your Calorie intake by 3,500 a week, and you'll lose a pound. What should your own individual calorie intake be? Write down your desirable weight (take the weight in the middle of your weight range for your height)—the one you'd really feel you should be to be both healthy and look good. Multiply this by 15, then subtract 500. For instance, if your ideal weight is 125 pounds, you multiply that by 15, get 1,875, subtract 500—and come up with a permissible Calorie intake of 1375.

Of course, different people have different calorie needs. Recommended calorie intake is affected by many variables including size and sex, basal metabolism, climate, but mostly by physical activity. All individuals are different, but each person can estimate his own requirements with the help of his scale, a tape measure, and, if need be, his physician.

Activities vary in the number of calories they require and hence use up. Sitting or studying uses up 28 Calories in an hour; dishwashing and ironing will burn up 70. Walking requires 140, running

490, and bicycling 530. It all depends on what you do and how you do it.

Foods vary in the calories they provide. Your chart may say that a medium-sized apple has 70 Calories. But this does not mean that the apple you are eating has 70 Calories. It may have 50 or 60. Your chart may state that an "average" serving of roast beef is 250 Calories. What you had for Sunday dinner could have been less, or more.

Eyes and guesses vary. A big problem in counting calories is *you*, and what you think you eat, and when, and how. What is medium to you is large, or small, to your neighbor. An egg is an egg, but is it boiled or fried or scrambled? Did you eat your meat fat or cut it off? Did you use or omit gravy and sauce, and butter on your vegetable? Was your teaspoon of sugar for the coffee scant or heaping? Did you count the cocktail before dinner, and the crackers that went with it, the snack you had with coffee, the beer while you watched TV?

Yes, there are variations, and complications. Still, you can have your fun and your food and your liquid refreshment if you just remember one cardinal principle: Cut down, not out. Moderation in food, moderation in drink, and moderation in activity: these are three vital keys to health and a good weight.

You need not go to extremes of starvation, and you need not hike fifty miles.

To be effective, a diet must be a permanent design for living, and must include all the essential nutrients for health; it must also include foods that an individual likes and enjoys, and that are easily obtained and fit into the budget. The diet must not be punishing. Fast weight loss by rigid restriction is useless, because the pounds pile up again. Slow and steady is the way to win this race.

Here Are the Specifics

Enough philosophy. Here are some specific tips for losing some of the extra weight you are carrying around with you.

Tip 1. Think about what you ate and drank yesterday—and the day before that. Make a list of everything you consumed, and the approximate portions. Don't limit yourself to the three meals you ate—but list all snacks, samples, and nibbles. Be honest! Get a detailed calorie counter and calculate your caloric Bottom Line.

How much over your ideal is it? Consider, for instance, this fairly typical too-high-in calories menu. Does this look anything like your current one?

Breakfast	*Calories*
Orange juice—4 ounces	55
Cereal—1 serving	105
Milk—1 cup	165
Toast or plain roll—1	75
Jelly—1 tsp.	55
Coffee—2 cups, with 1 tsp. sugar and 1 tsp. milk	50
Total Calories for breakfast	505

Midmorning "Coke"	78

Lunch	*Calories*
Bouillon or clear soup	25
Cold chicken sandwich, with butter or mayonnaise	275
Lettuce and tomato salad—no dressing	25
Strawberry shortcake—no cream	347
Iced tea—sugar and lemon	15
Total Calories for lunch	687

Afternoon Snack	
Dish of chocolate ice cream	270

Dinner	*Calories*
Martinis—2 (each 2 ounces of gin)	420
Tomato juice cocktail	35
Broiled halibut—with lemon and 1 pat butter	205
Parsley potato	100
French-style green beans	35
Roll—1	75
Margarine—1 pat	50
Jelly—1 tsp.	55
Grapefruit-orange salad—no dressing	45
Jello—no cream	65
Tea—1 cup, with sugar and lemon	15
Total Calories for dinner	1100

Bedtime Snack

Beer (12 ounces) and 4 pretzels	190
Total Calories for the day	2830

For you, 2830 Calories may well be too many. Now consider some specific suggestions on cutting those calories back, say to 2200, without starving or punishing yourself:

Calories Saved

1. Reduce the martinis to 1, or use only
   1 ounce of gin in each   210

2. Omit the dessert at lunch   347

3. Omit the margarine at dinner or use diet soda
   for your midmorning snack   80

4. Omit sugar or milk from breakfast coffee   25

5. Instead of 3 and 4, have a dish of vanilla ice cream
   rather than chocolate ice cream   65

                         Total saving—approximately   600-700

OR

Omit about half of the calories suggested above and do forty-five minutes more per day of some type of brisk exercise—a fast walk will do. This type of approach to menu planning need not mean daily meal planning with an adding machine (or as one bitter dieter complained, "You've got to stop eating food and begin eating calories"). You should just check on your total intake occasionally and, if necessary, think of ways of cutting calorie corners.

Tip 2. Make sure that you have a well-rounded, varied diet to provide the minerals, vitamins, and protein you need. Every day's meals should include one to two glasses of milk (skim for fewer calories) or cheese; meat, fish, poultry, or egg; four servings of fruits and vegetables, of which one should be citrus for vitamin C and one a dark-green or yellow vegetable for vitamin A; and some vitamin B-rich whole-grain or enriched bread or cereal. Don't skimp on the Basic Four!!

Then watch the luxury foods. This does not refer to cost, but to calories, and includes those delicious but disastrous dishes that pile on the pounds: fried and fatty foods, hot rolls and biscuits, sauces, salad dressings, desserts, and even extra bread. Count the soft drinks, beer, and cocktails too, and all the tempting tidbits that accompany them. Alcohol, particularly, can play tricks on you. It supplies 7 Calories per gram, which means that one ounce of gin averages 105 Calories. It may not look like that many, but take our word for it, they are all there! Since no one has yet come up with a low-calorie alcohol, serious weight watchers must choose between dessert or a cocktail—not both. A word on the way alcohol can trick you. If you have a few drinks one night and then step on the scale the next day, you are deluding yourself if you think the weight loss you see is real. Actually you are seeing the effects of dehydration—and thirst will soon take care of that.

Tip 3. Cut corners cleverly. Make your meals attractive. Avoid skipping or skimping some meals, which leads to overeating at others. And when you open the refrigerator at snack time for "a bite," keep these sample figures in mind.

"Just a little sandwich" (hamburger on a bun)	330 Calories
Chocolate malted milk	500 Calories
Pumpkin pie with whipped cream	460 Calories
Small chocolate nut sundae with whipped cream	400 Calories
Cream puff	450 Calories
Mincemeat pie serving	400 Calories

Tip 4. Don't cut out foods—particularly those you like. *Cut down on them.* Put your meals on a small plate. You won't feel sorry for yourself then—and when you finish everything there, chances are you'll be just as satisfied as you would be from a larger amount. Eat slowly too. That should help cut down on your total intake.

Tip 5. Consider some psychological aids. Dr. Theodore Isaac Rubin, a formerly fat psychiatrist, suggests that you think of your favorite fattening foods as poisons. Look at that piece of chocolate cream pie and imagine it comes complete with a skull and crossbones.

Or maybe you could put a picture of yourself on the refrigerator with the caption, "Think Less of Me." Maybe it would help if you told all your friends you were dieting so you would have their teasing to worry about if you go off the diet. For you it might be useful to begin your diet on a birthday, an anniversary, after a big holiday—or on a Monday morning. Fine. But remember that the more you put it off, the more you put it on.

Tip 6. Beware of the diet saboteur. Dr. Wilmer L. Asher, executive director of the American Society of Bariatric Physicians (weight control doctors) has pointed out that dieters are often surrounded by anti-diet advice from "concerned friends." Be prepared for those who try to tempt you with appealing foods or make a great show of how they are enjoying their calorie-filled meals or disparage your need to lose weight. It's possible they are simply jealous of your intentions—or fear that your personality or attitude toward them might change once you have slimmed down.

Tip 7. Beware of too much relaxation or too much rigidity. Small indulgences can pack a big calorie wallop; on the other hand, to err occasionally is not fatal—it's human.

When you eat with moderation, the life you save may be your own. When you lead the way for your family, the life you save may be your child's.

MORE TIPS: READ THOSE ADS CAREFULLY

What you don't know *can* hurt you. What's left unsaid in ads is often more important than what is actually told. As the Romans would say, *"Caveat lector"*—let the reader beware.

Food processors advertise, like most other people, for the plain and simple reason that they want to sell more of their product. Naturally they want their advertising agency to design ads that make their products more attractive and desirable than those of their competitors. It's the American way.

If you're determined to be a wise shopper, read between the lines!

For example, are you trying to find an easy way to shed unwanted adiposity? If so, keep a level and analytical head on your shoulders when you see ads that announce joyfully, "You can use ———— like ———— and get only half as many fat calories." Or "Use ————, it has half the fat calories of ————."

True, the advertised product will have less fat and fewer calories, just as the ads say.

Take plain yogurt. Some kinds may have only half the fat content of whole milk and therefore half as many fat calories. But here's the catch. We get calories not only from the fat in food, but also from the carbohydrate and protein in them. These are the facts you're not told about. The Calories add up to 125 for a cup of this type of yogurt and 170 for the whole milk. Less, but not half! Yogurt does have half the fat calories of milk and fewer total calories. It is an excellent food, as are all milk products.

Exactly the same type of advertising has been used for many other food products—for example, evaporated milk with "half the fat calories." This is not the same as "half the total calories."

Then some bread companies advertise a so-called "low-calorie" bread, designed to aid the weight watchers. The ads will say that such and such a bread is high in protein, vitamins and minerals, "yet only has 46 Calories per 18-gram slice." This claim is true and unless you are pretty well informed you might think that this is really a calorie-saving product. Your calorie booklet says that a slice of regular bread supplies 60 Calories. Here is where you need to think. Slices of most regular breads weigh from 23 to 25 grams each. Trim 5 or 6 grams off your slice of regular bread and you have an 18-gram slice furnishing 46 Calories. The "special" bread is either sliced thinner, or the loaf is smaller in diameter than the conventional one.

So be a wise shopper; pay attention to the "ads." This is one way to keep up to date with new products and processes. But be sure you read with understanding; that when you hear, you also listen; that when you look, you see. Those "ads" are probably truthful, but they may not say what you think they do.

Nutritional labeling is a big help here because if food manufacturers are to push the nutritional qualities of their products, they must state the calorie value of a defined serving.

And Still More: Tips on the Timing of Food

Another fringe benefit resulting from some interesting research that can be used to advantage has to do with when and how we eat.

You can lose weight by eating and gain weight by not eating.

Does that sound absurd? It isn't really. The answer is in the timing of food intake.

Food consumed thirty to sixty minutes before a meal tends to dull the appetite and thus lessen the desire for a large meal. Therefore, fat people who wish to lose weight might well have a snack before a meal and then be satisfied with a smaller meal. But they should not by any means consider the snack a token and then consume the regular portions that contributed to their obesity in the first place.

Thin people trying to gain weight should avoid a snack before meals. They want a good appetite at mealtime. They should have their snack afterward in order to pack in some extra calories.

As with most other things, timing is important. Take medicines, for example. They are most effective when taken on an empty stomach. That is when they are most quickly absorbed.

Vitamins or food supplements, on the other hand, deliver their greatest benefits when taken with meals. There is a good reason for this. Most of the water-soluble vitamins such as vitamin C or those of the B complex are quickly eliminated by the body in the urine. If they are taken between meals they will be gone by the time of the next meal when they should be present along with the carbohydrate, protein, and fat of the food in order to help utilize or metabolize these three major sources of energy.

It is extremely important that supplements of amino acids be taken with meals. All essential amino acids must be present in the blood at about the same time for efficient protein utilization.

This has been shown clearly in studies with ordinary breakfast cereals. When they were consumed dry, or with water, and the milk taken a few hours later, the nutritional effect was not as pronounced as when the milk was consumed with the cereal.

Why? Because some of the amino acids from the incomplete cereal protein had passed through the body before the missing amino acids of the milk were supplied. This is also why nibbling or snacking, especially if the snacks are "unscientific" or "empty" calorie ones, often contribute little to our nutritional state, but a lot to our overweight state.

Good News for Nibblers

Nibbling isn't entirely bad.

But wait! This doesn't mean you can go hog-wild. Do not confuse controlled nibbling with free-lance snacking.

Calories still have to be considered, despite what you may have read in a best-selling book. Total calories consumed in a day have to add up to fewer than calories used for energy to lose weight, and more to gain weight. The day's food must supply the day's requirements of some fifty nutrients.

It's possible, though, that if the food is nibbled frequently, consumed in several more or less equal portions throughout the day, this may be an improvement over our present system. Meal eating is a matter of custom and convenience, and perhaps our patterns need some rearranging.

Mealtimes and places and amounts have changed through the decades. Breakfast, lunch and dinner foods and menus vary in different lands, in different climates, and with different occupations.

Generally speaking, before the era of the seven or eight-hour day, workers rose with the dawn and sweated long past sunset. Plenty of food was needed to support this labor, and nearly everyone had frequent hearty meals.

Things are different now. Breakfast is frequently a hurry-up fruit-juice-and-coffee affair, with lunch a quick bite sandwiched into a fast half-hour. The dinner accounts for the lion's share of the day's nutrition. There's a big slab of meat covered with gravy and accompanied by potatoes and vegetables. There's bread and margarine too, and dessert and beverage. If all this is preceded by cocktails or followed by liqueurs, still more is crammed into the stomach. So most of the eating occurs in one short part of the day, and in the part of the day when there's the least activity.

Recent experiments suggest that this pattern of two skimpy snack-type meals followed by a bang-up binge at dinner is not a good idea, particularly in the absence of exercise. Perhaps nibbling, or at least a better distribution of food and activity, is better for health.

Work with laboratory animals suggests that consideration should be given not only to what is eaten but also to how and when food is eaten.

Chickens, for example, even when they don't have to pick and peck in the barnyard for their daily food, seem to thrive better when they eat in dribs and drabs. Doctors in Chicago did studies in which chickens were divided into two similar groups. One had free access to food, while the second was fed just once daily. Those in the second group showed more evidence of atherosclerosis, the condition found in humans with heart disease, than did the nibbling chicks.

It is also pertinent that eating habits are often very different in the countries where heart disease is not the serious problem that it is in the United States. The wait-and-gorge-at-dinner custom that stamps this country contrasts strikingly with the more evenly balanced pattern in many other nations.

It will be interesting to see what further nutrition experiments disclose. Meanwhile, observations suggest that with regard to meals, as well as choice of foods, the wise person is the moderate person. Part of being wise is being informed and discriminating. And part of successful dieting is increased calorie expenditure—otherwise known as exercise.

FIRST AID WITH EXERCISE

A calorie countdown is the beginning of wisdom, especially when it is combined with an exercise upswing. Too much food and too little exercise are wreaking havoc in the United States these days.

Creeping obesity is a specter that haunts us all. Even at the age of twenty-five, body energy needs begin to diminish. By the forties and fifties caloric requirement is reduced by 10 percent; this decreases to as much as 30 percent by the seventies. Yet appetites do not work the same way. Waistlines widen because appetites outstrip caloric needs.

While we are constantly tempted by calories, we avoid the activity that would help us burn up some of the extra calories. Ours is a land of automation and automobiles, of buses, planes, and escalators. Hikes have gone out of style, and golf carts have taken the walking even out of golf. We have abandoned the horse and buggy but not the food habits of those bygone years. We eat as much, or more, while we move less and less.

Yet exercise is important. It takes away fat and flabbiness. Moderate and regular exercise does not increase the appetite, and it burns up extra calories.

Are you surprised to hear that exercise does not increase your appetite? The human body has an appetite regulating mechanism. It is when we become sedentary that this mechanism fails to operate properly. When we are moving around as we were meant to, we don't have to worry so much about overeating. Again, experiments at Harvard's nutrition department have shown that rats that exercised one or two hours a day did not eat more than the non-exercising rats. In fact they ate less. This observation is nothing new to animal raisers: farmers have long known about this and make sure they pen up any animals they wish to fatten.

Now we *are* in favor of exercise—but don't get carried away with the idea that if you keep active and busy then calories don't count. They still do. For instance, you've probably heard a stout friend of yours (if you haven't said it yourself) say, "Oh, I'll walk it off . . ." as he takes another helping of a rich dessert. Just to give you an idea of what type of walking would be necessary, consider the chart below.

The "Oh, I'll Walk It Off" Table

If You Eat . . .	*These Many Miles Will "Walk It Off". . .*
One piece of chocolate cake with icing	5.3 miles
1 piece of mince pie	4.5 miles
1 doughnut	3.7 miles
1 ice cream cone	3.1 miles
1 ten-ounce can of beer	2.2 miles

Would you walk 5.3 miles for a piece of cake? Well, you could say that was a matter of opinion. But the point here is not to denigrate exercise as a means of keeping your weight where you want it to be, but to emphasize that exercise and calorie control must go together. We've heard people say, "Oh, I'd have to ride my bike 7½ hours after dinner to use up the number of calories I need to. It's not worth it!" But there's another way of looking at it: if you take a half-hour bike ride every night you could shed twenty-six pounds in a year.

What kind of exercise is best? The kind you do yourself! Massages, steam baths, and health machines may make you feel fine, but they won't keep the weight off. They mostly reduce your wallet.

It *does* help to push away from the table before the seconds are passed around. And another very effective table exercise involves vigorously shaking your head from side to side when you're offered rich desserts. Most effective of all is conscientious adherence to a planned program—day-to-day conditioning and reconditioning.

There is a big difference between those who sit and those who move. Often the contrast between fat and thin people is not so much what they eat, but what they do and how they do it.

Exercise is without doubt a must for firm muscles and figure control. And exercise brings big fringe benefits too. You will not only look better, you will *be* better, and you will feel better.

It is no surprise to hear that exercise is good for your health. Exercise promotes the growth of collateral blood vessels which may take over if there is any narrowing in the main coronary vessels feeding the heart. People who take the time to exercise generally live longer. A classic British study showed that London bus drivers had a higher incidence and greater severity of coronary heart disease than did bus conductors. If you have ever been on a British bus, you know that the conductors must run up and down between the two levels collecting tolls. They get exercise! Of course, there remains the possibility that the bus drivers were under more stress—because of traffic conditions or disagreeable passengers—and that may have led them to have more heart trouble; but coupled with other evidence we have about the role exercise plays in promoting health, the first conclusion seems more likely.

Reflections on Dieting

Humorist Art Buchwald has described his many attempts at dieting. He explains that the first day is always fine—he only faints twice, and he manages to get through it by going to bed by eight o'clock. Buchwald concluded that the first week of a diet is particularly rough, but the second is very easy, primarily because the odds are that you are off it by then.

Another perpetually dieting comedian, San Levenson, who complains, "I never met a crumb I didn't like," and laments that he used to think calories were holes in the teeth, has also written a great deal about dieting philosophy. He has described the travails of having to approach food with a tape measure (white fish, steamed, 4" x 4" x ¾") and odd serving containers ("one cup of liver," "three tablespoons of pistachios") and rues the hunger that inevitably follows gourmet diet dishes. (The recipe for one such dish, marinated mushrooms, was "scrub one mushroom, peel it, soak it in thorns vinaigrette, and stew it in a thimble".) He finally reached the conclusion that the only way to manage on a diet is to gulp down all the rich foods you see so you won't be tempted to eat them later.

Anyone who has tried to lose weight quickly through semi-starvation understands what Buchwald and Levenson are talking about. It is true that the average diet does much for the willpower and so little for the waistline. Why? Because too many people approach dieting in an unrealistic manner. They want results right away—and they look forward to a quick return to their normal intake of excess calories. It takes weeks, months to put on weight; it will take equally as long to take it off. Dieting should not be a question of starving yourself so you can live longer. It need not take the starch out of you if you approach it scientifically and patiently—and make a lifelong philosophy out of eating and drinking moderately. And if you are patient about seeing results. Remember, if at first you don't recede, diet, diet again.

FAD DIETS DON'T WORK

Perhaps the most lucrative of the food faddist's endless supply of moneymaking compounds are the get-thin-quick concoctions.

When you go into a bookstore these days, you find about as many diet books as there are calories in Boston cream pie. Volumes offering diet and nutrition advice are now outselling those offering counsel about sex. Weight reduction has become a national pastime, given that most American eaters are aware of the health risks which go with obesity—increased risks of diabetes, diseases of the heart, liver, kidney and blood vessels, high blood pressure—and they are highly motivated to shed their excess adipose.

Their uselessness has been discovered by hundreds of disappointed dieters, all of whom unfailingly regain weight as soon as they abandon the fad-of-the-month. Unfortunately, however, year after creative year, reducing foods, fads, formulas and pills continue to enrich their ingenious promoters.

There is no magic in low or high carbohydrate, low or high fat, grapefruit or bananas or eggs. There is absolutely no scientific basis for any drastic juggling of food constituents. The two-fold result is an unbalanced diet, which can be damaging if it is prolonged, and a ceaseless process of losing and gaining, which is as undesirable as it is frustrating.

There is also no such thing as "fattening" or "slimming" foods,

or magic reducing foods. Patients have to learn, unpleasant though
the lesson may be, that excess weight is simply an inevitable result
of excess calorie intake and that calories count, whether they come
from carbohydrate or fat or protein, from bread or bourbon or beef
or blueberries. The only way to get slim is to eat less and to exercise more. The only way to stay slim is to form new habits of eating
with moderation and exercising with vigor, and to keep this up forever!

The wishbone, however, is stronger than the backbone; so it is a
tough assignment to outdo the tempting salesmen who blandly
promise miracles. The public health profession can only win this
battle of wits if it recognizes the strength of the adversary and
resolves to act promptly, forcefully and cleverly.

With tricks adapted from the quack and tools borrowed from the
educator, professional workers can make sense as attractive as nonsense. Let the truth be glamorized and used to expose the fraud in
all the false promises that sell false cures!

For their own devious purposes the faddists have been exploiting a
widespread interest in nutrition and health. Now it is time for the
bona fide health worker to capitalize on this concern and to convince the quack's clientele that rejection of today's foods and today's
physicians in favor of old-fashioned fads and slippery salesmen is
utterly foolish. It is as senseless as substitution of a horse and
buggy for the automobile. Look at some specifics. We won't have to
go far to find some examples. Your local newstand with its various
popular magazines will give you a taste of the diet craze.

In any month one can be sure to find a new diet advertised on the
front of magazines, diets guaranteed to succeed where others have
failed. Consider just a few of the diets randomly picked from recent
women's magazines:

The Grapefruit Diet	Mother and Daughter Diet
No-Hunger Rice Diet	Meat and Mushroom Diet
Egg and Wine Diet	New Natural Foods Reducing Diet
Pumpkin and Carrot Diet	Your Personalized Computer Diet
Debutante Diet	The No-Willpower Diet
Champagne Diet	How to Eat Everything and
After-Divorce Diet	Lose Weight

The fact that there are so many diets might suggest to you immediately the obvious fact that if one of them worked, there would

be no need each month to come up with a new one. But the fact remains that each year countless articles and books are written— and many of the books find their way to the top of the best-seller list. Overweight is big business!

The shortcomings and hazards of the diets we hear about most often deserve particular attention. Let's start with the age-old low-carbohydrate diets which have appeared cyclically every few years wrapped in a new package and bearing a new author's name.

The Low-Carbohydrate Diets

You'll see this diet recently sold under the name *Dr. Atkins' Diet Revolution* (by R. C. Atkins) or *The Doctor's Quick Weight Loss Diet* (I. M. Stillman and S. S. Baker). But don't think these are new. As we mentioned earlier, these low-carbohydrate diets, now being sold as "revolutionary," are neither new nor innovative. Recall that Dr. William Harvey wrote about this back in 1863—but at least he had an excuse because the basics of nutrition were unknown then.

Since the nineteenth century the low-carbohydrate diet has reappeared regularly—guaranteeing instant success and significant royalties for the author. In the last twenty-five years it has been sold under such titles as *Calories Don't Count, The Drinking Man's Diet, The Air Force Diet* and others. Remember, these are all basically the same; they have been tried for over a century without results. But authors and publishers keep reselling this "magic formula" and gullible would-be dieters eagerly consume it and continue to put on weight.

1. The Atkins Diets: "Super Energy" and "The Diet Revolution"

You can eat as much bacon, heavy cream cheese, mayonnaise, marbled steak, egg dishes as you want and still—miraculously—lose weight.

So says Dr. Robert C. Atkins in his books describing variations of the so-called "Atkins Diet." But you must strictly avoid foods containing sugars and starch. How does such a menu lead to a slimmer you? According to Dr. Atkins, when you eat no carbohydrates, your body produces a "fat mobilizing hormone" which converts it from a carbohydrate-burning engine into a fat-burning one. This appealing theory was set forth in *Dr. Atkins' Diet Revolu-*

tion. And the new "Super Energy Diet" merely extends his original ideas to include vitamin supplements and offers twists on this diet theory to accommodate those who are trying to maintain weight, put on weight or cope with excess pounds during special circumstances like pregnancy.

Does the diet work? Do you lose weight and keep it off? Unfortunately, the answer to both questions is "no." There is simply no way that you can ingest four to five thousand Calories a day—no matter what the source—and shed pounds. The fats which are recommended on the Atkins diet contain nine Calories per gram as do all fats. Ironically, the carbohydrates that are strictly forbidden contain but four Calories per gram. If you religiously follow the Atkins "Revolutionary" plan you may notice an initial weight loss. This, however, can be traced primarily to loss of body water (a condition which temporarily makes the scale indicator sway toward the left)—and to the reality that diets free of all carbohydrates can get pretty boring, and you'll inevitably take in fewer calories.

Studies have shown that people on low-carbohydrate diets consume 13-15 percent fewer calories than they usually would. This would be a good path to weight control except in this case the calories taken in are not nutritionally balanced.

When thirst makes up for the dehydration and the dieter gets tired of a boring menu and returns to his regular overeating, any weight loss returns, and rather quickly.

But of more concern than the deceiving temporary weight loss are the health threatening side effects that accompany a no-carbohydrate routine. Carbohydrates are vital to any well-balanced diet. They provide the "brain food" we all need. When we deprive ourselves of them we experience headache, weakness—anything *but* super energy! Beyond that, the Atkins plan leads to an increased consumption of foods which are high in saturated fats and cholesterol, an immediate danger for anyone with a tendency toward heart disease and a generally undesirable pattern for anyone who is interested in promoting "heart health." Studies have documented a 16 percent or greater increase in blood cholesterol levels in a group of healthy young individuals on a high-protein, low-carbohydrate diet. According to AMA's spokesman, Dr. C. F. Butterworth, "The full impact [of this type of diet] may not become apparent to an individual's health until many years later." If that isn't enough to convince you that the Atkins diet is not for you, keep in mind that a low-carbohydrate intake favors an increase in blood uric acid which can exacerbate gout and simultaneously puts an extra burden on the kidneys.

High fat and low carbohydrates trigger an abnormal body response called ketosis, the increased production of ketones, usually associated with conditions of impaired metabolism such as diabetes.

Most immediately relevant to the majority of us, people on a low-carbohydrate diet complain of fatigue after a few days, a complaint characterized by a lack of energy for the normal activities of the day. These symptoms are the body's reaction to an imbalanced diet and can mean trouble. One advocate of a low-carbohydrate diet found this out the hard way.

On a television show in Houston, a diet faddist was debating with a physician who was concerned about the current preoccupation of Americans with low-carbohydrate diet books. The faddist remained staunch in his support of the regimen. The next morning, however, the physician received an emergency call from the dieter who explained that while he was rising from his morning bath, he blacked out, struck his head on the tub and nearly drowned. What had happened? The victim of diet faddism had suffered a dramatic drop in blood pressure when he shifted from the supine to the standing position. Any low-carbohydrate dieter understands this sense of dizziness upon rising. It results from the fact that the brain temporarily lacks sufficient blood to sustain consciousness.

The Council on Foods and Nutrition of the American Medical Association has reviewed the various low-carbohydrate diets that have come along and has expressed concern about them. Specifically commenting on the Atkins diet, the Council concluded that "the rationale advanced to justify the diet is, for the most part, without scientific merit . . . ." Furthermore, the Council was deeply concerned "about any diet that advocates 'unlimited' intake of saturated fats and cholesterol-rich foods." Finally, the medical group noted that "it is unfortunate that no reliable mechanism exists to help the public evaluate and put into proper perspective the great volume of nutritional information and misinformation with which it is constantly being bombarded . . . . Bizarre concepts of nutrition and dieting should not be promoted to the public as if they were established scientific principles. If appropriate precautions are not taken, information about nutrition and diet that is not only misleading but potentially dangerous to health will continue to be conveyed to the public."

2. The Stillman Diet

The late Dr. Irving Stillman in his book *The Doctor's Quick Weight Loss Diet* (and the follow-up versions, *The Doctor's Inches Off Diet, Quick Weight Loss Diet Cookbook, Teenage Diet*) advised a daily intake composed mainly of lean meat, poultry, lean fish, eggs and low-fat cheeses. You can eat as much of these foods as you wish —and, in addition you're required to drink at least eight glasses of water a day. The diet purports to burn up 275 more Calories a day than meals having the same calorie content but including carbohydrates and fats.

The Stillman approach, like the Atkins one, is basically a low-carbohydrate diet and has all the problems and risks that go with that. The "theory" behind it is nonsense and defies the basic law of thermodynamics, namely that energy does not just disappear. If you want to lose weight, you've got to eat fewer calories—or burn up more. Follow-up studies of those following Dr. Stillman's advice report fatigue, lassitude, mild nausea, occasional diarrhea—some symptoms being so serious that they interfered with work performance. The simplest nutritional analysis of the Stillman menu points to shortages of a number of vital body nutrients—carbohydrates, calcium, iron and some vitamins. The verdict on the Stillman diet is the same as for the Atkins diet: forget it.

Other Diet Nonsense

The Last Chance Diet

If cutting back a bit on what you normally eat is good, then cutting out *all* of what you normally eat must be better. So goes the philosophy of the Last Chance Diet, as summarized in a book of that name by Dr. Robert Linn, an osteopath who describes himself as "specializing in the practice of bariatric medicine." Dr. Linn calls for the total elimination of food for one or more months. The only thing he allows his weight-conscious followers is a substance called "Prolinn" which he claims ". . . is one of the best protein sources . . . ." It is not. It is one of the poorest protein sources. It is a chemical digest of one of the poorest proteins, collagen, which is scraped or "cooked" from animal hides before they are made into leather. It doesn't begin to compare in nutritional quality to the protein of eggs, milk, meat, poultry, or fish. We don't know of a worse protein than collagen.

Further, it is utterly ridiculous to have any protein "pre-digested" because several body tissues, particularly the pancreas, are regular "enzyme factories" that efficiently and effectively "digest" our foods, including protein.

When you are on the Last Chance Diet, you get to have a few tablespoons of this cherry-flavored nonsensical potion each day plus vitamin and mineral supplements—and that's all. Total caloric intake may approximate 300-400 Calories. Who wouldn't lose weight on such a caloric intake? Dr. Linn feels that this protein supplement offers a diet (?) with the advantage of a total fast but approximates the protein requirement so that the majority of what is lost from the body during the fast is fat, not protein.

Starvation diets have a place in diet therapy but only in the most unique circumstances—and only under strict medical supervision, almost always in a hospital. When you deny yourself food for long periods of time, your body must undergo radical changes to cope with the absence of food. For example, glycogen reserves in the liver must be converted to make available the necessary amounts of essential glucose. Body potassium and sodium are quickly lost. The body develops a state of ketosis, and then acidosis, a situation where uric acid levels in the blood become very high, favoring, as we already mentioned, the development of diseases such as gout. No amount of a poor protein supplement is going to keep body metabolism on an even keel while you starve yourself and lose weight. Thus, in following the Last Chance Diet, you would essentially be trying to run a complex machine without the necessary type of fuel. The several deaths that have been reported among those using liquid, predigested protein diets, and the activities of the FDA bear witness to the extreme hazards of this reducing nonsense.

Unless your obesity condition requires drastic, medically supervised action, starvation is not the way to lose weight. And it certainly is not a practical way of maintaining weight. Coming to terms with a weight problem means adjusting your food intake, learning to live with less but proper food, not without it.

Dr. Frank's No Aging Diet: Eat and Grow Younger

Dr. Benjamin S. Frank claims to have written the first diet book to be based on the scientific breakthrough (naturally!) of our times. By eating foods rich in nucleic acids, that is, those rich in RNA and DNA, you will cause every cell in your body to become young again. Basically what Dr. Frank is offering is a dietary Fountain of Youth.

The Frank formula for growing younger is a massive network of scientific gobbledygook which calls for eating lots of sardines (a three or four-ounce can at least four days a week), and adding generous amounts of calves' liver, beets, soybeans and lentils to fill in the other days' fare. The simple theory presented to explain his recommendations is that since nucleic acids RNA and DNA are scientifically accepted as the fundamental genetic material that determines the essential makeup of each living creature, we can stay healthier and resist aging by eating from this rich source.

Of course, there is no scientific evidence that our bodies benefit from extra dietary nucleic acids (the body regularly produces them anyway), because in the process of digestion they are destroyed and broken down to simpler chemical compounds. The diet itself, unless you happen to be enamored of sardines, is very limited and rather high in salt content, high levels of sodium presenting special dangers in hypertension.

The HCG Diet

This diet in the western part of the U.S. generally goes under the name "Simeon Weight Reduction" program. In the East, the focal points of the movement are the "Kennedy Diet Centers," which are concentrated in the New York area, but have spread to the Midwest as well. In both cases, the HCG diet calls for a 500 Calorie a day intake plus regular shots of the hormone HCG, short for human chorionic gonadotropin, a hormone which is extracted from the urine of pregnant women.

British-born physician Dr. Albert T. Simeon used the hormone in the treatment of young boys suffering from a condition known as Froehlich's syndrome. Injections of HCG helped reduce the accumulation of fat on the hips, buttocks and thighs which made such boys look like girls. The hormone seemed to "melt away" the feminizing fat, so Dr. Simeon and his followers reasoned that with the liberated fat as a major source of nourishment, would-be dieters could benefit from the drug.

Basically the Simeon-Kennedy Center diets are semi-starvation regimens combined with a psychological boost of daily visits to a clinic. Side effects of HCG therapy include headache, restlessness, depression—but more important are the unknown, possibly long-term, effects of exposure to such a potent hormone. Studies by the Food and Drug Administration concluded that "there are no scientifically adequate, well-controlled clinical studies appearing in medical literature which establish the safety and efficiency of HCG in the treatment of obesity." HCG injections do have a place in medical therapy (in addition to being used in Froehlich's syndrome, HCG is often helpful in treating infertility in women) but, again, common sense would tell you that the use of such a drug where it has no known beneficial effect is not smart.

The Pritikin Diet

Nathan Pritikin, Director of the Longevity Research Institute in Santa Barbara, California, recently made headlines in the popular press when he claimed that he could cure heart disease by putting patients on fat-restricted diets. The implication of his theory is that you can similarly *prevent* heart disease and live a long happy life if you follow a nearly fat-free menu.

Certainly most all nutritionists now ageee that American diets are too rich in fat, particularly saturated fat, and that we'd be healthier if we cut our intake from 40 percent down to about 30 percent of total calories. But the menus that Mr. Pritikin has in mind (he permits only 10 percent of calories to be fat) make the American Heart Association menu look like a Roman banquet. The Pritikin diet allows turkey, fish, fruits (but only four pieces a day), sourdough bread, rice, pasta and skimmed dairy products, but expressly forbids all butter, margarine, oil, grain-fed beef, sugar and products containing these ingredients.

The intent of the Pritikin plan is admirable, but its extremism is unrealistic. Not only is it for most people an almost impossible diet to live with—severely limiting your choice of food—but there is no scientific evidence that such drastic cutback in fat is necessary or desirable. You cannot undo the effects of years of overeating by restricting fat intake for one or two months (and it is unlikely that you would stick with this diet much longer than this). If you are worried about eating too much fat (and if you are like the typical

American, you probably *have reason* to worry), try a more moderate, but long-term cutback of rich foods.

The Save Your Life Diet

Dr. David Rubin claims that if you add significant amounts of fiber to your diet, you will protect yourself from a number of the most serious diseases which affect Americans today, including cancer of the colon and diseases of the heart.

He based his conclusions on the work of some British investigators (including Drs. Denis Burkitt and Hugh Trowel) who observed that the incidence of these afflictions was lower in developing countries in Africa than it was in Western countries—and that the key element seemed to be that Americans eat an overprocessed, low-fiber diet, one which slows the movement of food through the intestines, leading to relatively small, hard, dry stools, raising blood cholesterol levels.

As we mentioned in chapter four, information about the role of fiber in disease prevention is still being accumulated, but at least one conclusion is in: bran and related foods do *not* constitute the "save your life" diet. Certainly high-in-fiber foods are a pleasant and nutritious contribution to a well-balanced diet and, if you have a problem with constipation, increasing fiber intake may be of benefit to you. The evidence linking high-fiber diets to low rates of colon cancer and heart disease are based on a limited number of statistical associations. Evidence from animal studies do not support the Rubin recommendations nor have studies of Americans on high-fiber diets ever shown that they develop these diseases with less frequency than do those following medium or low-fiber diets. Evidence of other health promoting benefits of bran simply have not reached the point where it is legitimate to recommend major changes in the U.S. diet. Again, the fiber idea is just that—an idea. The populations that Dr. Rubin points to in Africa may have lower incidence of the specific diseases he discusses, but we can't overlook the obvious fact that Americans, on the average, live much longer than the African groups. Of concern is the possible undesirable side effects of a marked increase in dietary fiber. For example, it is known that fiber can bind other nutrients in the intestines, that is, interfere with the ability of vital elements to perform their biological functions in the body. These and other issues need to be resolved before bran is advocated as the new path to health and longevity.

Dr. Siegal's Natural Fiber Permanent Weight Loss Diet

Taking the dietary fiber hypothesis one step further, Dr. Sanford Siegal claims that "unquestionably . . . fiber-free processed food . . . is the main cause of obesity in our society." His recommendation might be set to tune as "fiber in the morning, fiber at noon and in the evening, and fiber at supper time," the result, he claims, being rapid and permanent weight loss, as well as protection from coronary artery and colon diseases. When fiber is removed from your food, Dr. Siegal says, you are consuming nothing but "naked calories."

Again, despite the statements of both Drs. Rubin and Siegal, the "evidence" that fiber diets protect from heart disease is not available. Perhaps the important factor here is that individuals eating lots of fiber have less time and appetite for eating diets high in fat, and that it is low fat, not high fiber, that is good for your heart.

To call fiber a weight reduction aid is equally misleading. If you eat a great deal of bran cereal, whole-grain bread, it may take you longer to chew, and you'll leave the table having eaten less. Or you may find that high fiber food swells up your stomach, satisfying you to the extent that you'll turn down "seconds" and high calorie desserts. But in itself, fiber has no biological properties that promote weight loss.

The Crenshaw Super Diet

Include some kelp, lecithin, vitamin B_6 and cider vinegar at each meal, and this will be your natural way to super beauty and a slim trim figure, says author Mary Ann Crenshaw. She favors cider as a weight-loss, health-promoting food on the grounds that it has potassium (but she fails to note that half a grapefruit provides more than three times as much potassium). Her interest in kelp apparently is related to the fact that it contains iodide, and this might be a means of stimulating the thyroid, leading to stepped-up metabolism and subsequent weight loss. What she does not note is that by eating seafood or using iodized salt, the body gets all the iodide it needs. And eating excess amounts of this mineral, instead of stimulating the thyroid, can indeed depress it, slowing down the metabolism. Why is lecithin included? This natural emulsifier, she says, is "full of Vitamin E, the sexy shaper-upper," a claim that has absolutely no scientific basis. This last "miracle food" is included to help "burn the fat away," a very strange conclusion, given that vitamin B_6, also known as pyridoxine, functions primarily in the metabolism of protein, not fat.

Interestingly, Ms. Crenshaw, who is neither a nutritionist nor a physician, also recommends that her magic formula (which is generally available in so-called health-food stores in one large capsule) be used in conjunction with a low-calorie diet. It should be no surprise, then, that it can work!

The Mayo Diet

This diet has appeared under a number of names—"the grapefruit diet" or "the egg and bacon diet." Presumably one can eat all the grapefruit, eggs and bacon one desires and yet lose weight. It is claimed that grapefruit contains enzymes which get rid of calories by speeding up the burning of body fat. Thus you are to start each meal with a grapefruit; the rest of the meal, as well as any snacks, must be only eggs and bacon, as much as you can eat—as long as you have your grapefruit.

A grapefruit is a perfectly useful and delicious food, but it is *not* a big yellow spark plug that ignites away your fat. Needless to say, the prestigious Mayo Clinic has nothing to do with this dietary nonsense and, indeed, the clinic has a strict low-calorie diet of its own which is based on sense, not nonsense.

The Zen-Macrobiotic Diet

This mixture of occultism, mysticism, religion and dietary extremism promises to cure all illness, past and present, improve memory and judgment, while at the same time "expanding freedom and thinking." Its name translates to a "long life"—but, indeed, should you actually follow it strictly, its effect will be exactly the opposite.

The Zen-Macrobiotic diet is actually ten diets, ranging from the lowest level which includes 10 percent cereals, 30 percent vegetables, 10 percent soup, 30 percent animal products, 15 percent salads and fruits and 5 percent desserts, to the highest which is 100 percent brown rice. Drastic restriction of all fluids is also recommended. Adherents believe that everything in the world is part of "yin" and "yang" and that healthy eating should offer a ratio of five yin to one yang. Sugar and most fruits are too yin and must be limited, meats and eggs are too yang. The only perfect food is brown rice. Tragically, a number of young Americans have followed this regimen, reaching the ultimate brown rice level and drastic restriction of fluids, and have lost their lives due to starvation and dehydration, apparently unaware that the diet is deficient in most vitamins, minerals and protein.

Surgical Diets

An English male nurse who weighed in at 322 pounds and whose normal daily diet included a whole chicken, four sandwiches, a pound of beef, dozens of slices of toast, a pound of chocolate, gallons of sweet coffee and tea, among other things, reportedly had his mouth clamped shut by a dental surgeon. For 112 days he sipped milk and lost 105 pounds.

With this report, a new diet technique was introduced: surgically locking the jaw, a technique normally used to treat a fractured jaw. Interestingly, a recent issue of the prestigious British medical publication *The Lancet* reported on the use of jaw-wiring in the treatment of obesity, noting "no major complications . . . patients tolerated the procedure and subsequent minor inconveniences." But the authors of the article also noted that two-thirds of the patients regained weight after the wires were removed.

As a weight reduction method, it appears that jaw-locking is nothing more than a gimmick—one which may well have hazards of its own. Locking your jaw can result in shifting the position of your teeth, can provoke gum disease and promote tooth decay, and poses the obvious danger that when the jaw is wired, what you cough or vomit may be inhaled directly into the lungs.

Another surgical gimmick involves what has come to be known as "staple-puncture," derived from the new interest in acupuncture, an ancient oriental art which involves inserting long needles into specific areas of the body for the purpose of killing pain or curing disease. On the assumption that there are "obesity nerve endings" in the ear, some weight reduction promoters have recommended surgical implantation of metal clips which dieters would wiggle when they felt hungry. Beyond serving as a reminder to stay on the 400-Calorie-a-day diet which accompanies this "treatment," the staple-puncture technique has been shown to have only one medical effect —it causes ear infections.

On a more drastic level is "dietary surgery," an operation technically known as jejuno-ileal bypass, where the intestines are severed at the jejunum and connected further down at the ileum. When food is eaten, it is poorly digested and only partly absorbed; thus the patient will lose weight.

The procedure has only been used on massively obese patients who, because of their weight, have their lives severely endangered. It is *not* a routine operation, by any means, and carries with it high risks of infection, liver failure and the formation of urinary stones.

Along the same lines, what has been described as "the diet to end all diets" is being tested at the University of Illinois. The basis for the weight loss regimen is a substance called perfluorooctyl bromide, a drug that coats the lining of the stomach and intestines to prevent food from being absorbed into the bloodstream. Allegedly, any food consumed while the drug is effective would then have the caloric impact of sawdust—and would ultimately be passed out of the body. The drug has so far only been tested on rats, but human trials are said to start soon. We doubt it!

The "Sex" Diet

Can sex keep you slim? Well, not really. But at least this diet won't hurt you!

The medical journal *Obesity and Bariatric Medicine* has calculated that if a person has sexual intercourse every day all year—everything else held constant—his body weight could be reduced by some six to nine pounds. This would involve a total energy expenditure of some fifty to seventy-five Calories, equivalent to a brisk walk on a level street or climbing one or two flights of stairs. Take your pick, but we suggest a combination!

"Minus Foods"

Can specific foods eaten before meals help you lose weight, and are there any "minus calorie foods"?

No and no. There are no "minus foods." This topic was given a great deal of attention a few years ago when a physician in Vienna claimed hard-cooked eggs, lean meat, some vegetables and fruits require so many elaborate chemical changes to digest them that they require more calories than they offer. Presumably if you followed the regimen of this diet you could arrange to disappear completely. But don't bother trying it. And when you see magazine articles (usually entitled something like "Eat, Eat, Eat Your Pounds Away"), turn the page.

DIET ORGANIZATIONS

If you need company to get your diet going, you have a number of organizations which are eager to offer it to you. Weight Watchers, TOPS (Take Off Pounds Sensibly) and the Diet Workshop are probably the best known ones.

Weight Watchers is a commercial corporation that requires weekly attendance, fees, and offers a rigidly structured diet, as well as lectures and social events. The rules are strict: no pills, no alcohol, no calorie counting, no substitution of the recommended foods, no meal skipping. The basic weight reduction diet calls for fish from a prescribed list of sixty "at least five times a week"; meat such as beef, lamb, three times a week; liver at least once; vegetables at lunch and dinner; fruits three to five times a day; a tablespoon of vegetable oil or two tablespoons of margarine a day; four eggs a week; skim milk; some cheese, bread or cereal; unlimited amounts of "legal" green vegetables such as celery and lettuce; moderate amounts of beans and tomatoes.

TOPS, which is probably the oldest of the self-help groups, in operation since 1952, offers its own set of guidance, separating men and women in its programs on the assumption that mixed company does not promote weight loss! Like Weight Watchers, it suggests medical supervision and is guided by general principles of good nutrition, including recommendations of the American Heart Association and American Diabetes Association regarding the use of fats and carbohydrates.

The Diet Workshop is the largest privately-owned franchised group weight control program. It was founded in Boston, Massachusetts, in 1965 by Lois L. Lindauer, the international director. After a successful first year of expansion in the Boston area, Ms. Lindauer opened in Springfield, Massachusetts. Later the Springfield groups were sold as a franchise, and The Diet Workshop was on the road to nationwide expansion.

There are now some sixty-seven franchises in thirty-one states, Canada, and Bermuda with over 1,900 groups containing approximately 50,000 people meeting weekly, and by the time this book is available undoubtedly there will be more.

The Diet Workshop program is a 1200-Calorie, measured-portion, three-meal-a-day balanced diet. In addition to stressing nutritional balance at mealtimes through the Basic Four foods, The Diet Workshop provides hints and tips on between-meal nibbles, snacks, and drinks that enable the dieters to be comfortably satiated while losing weight. Every week a new recipe is dictated to the class. Creative diet cooking is encouraged.

For the short run these self-help groups are reasonably successful, but the long-run success remains in question—but at least this type of dieting is not harmful to your health. If your diet needs moral support, and you can afford the fees for participation, it's worth a try.

The "Forget-It-All" Diets

And then there is the "to-hell-with-it diet," a philosophy you will find in books with a title which revolves around the theme "Fat Can Be Beautiful" and "Great Big Beautiful Doll." One of these books described the happiness of famous fatties and suggested that you too could be as happy as they if you stopped dieting and started living. One example offered was that of singer Cass Elliott, 5 feet 5½ inches tall, and 250 pounds. She was healthy, so why couldn't you be? Shortly after this particular book appeared, Miss Elliot was found dead in her London apartment, apparently a victim of a heart attack, at age thirty-three.*

Why the Fascination With Fad Diets?

People who desperately want to lose weight but refuse to read the "Basic Law of Calorie Intake and Expenditure" will believe anything.

When they see diets which encourage you to eat "juicy steaks and lobster swimming in butter," they are easy victims. They try it, see it doesn't work, stuff themselves to relieve their disappointment and then wait for the next fad diet to show up. Binge eating and binge dieting are not recommended. Mario Lanza ("the American Caruso"), who once enjoyed a twenty-three-egg omelet for breakfast,

---

*Ms. Elliott's death was originally attributed to choking on a sandwich, but later it was established that she had had a heart attack.

died of a heart attack at age thirty-eight after a lifetime of going on and off diets, once dropping 100 of his 270 pounds.

Do people have the right to write scientifically undocumented books and sell millions of copies which serve to mislead the public? Most definitely they do. It's their Constitutional right, and unless they do something illegal in the process no one will stop them. Indeed, television and radio talk show hosts will often encourage them to appear and bring the message—inaccurate and health threatening though it may be—to the public. When you see these individuals on TV and they appear glib and knowledgeable, keep in mind that these traits do not necessarily indicate the presence of nutritional know-how, they are just a part of the "show"!

Only once, as far as we know, did a temporary diet fad book run into legal problems. Dr. Herman Taller, author of *Calories Don't Count* (a variation of that old-fashioned low-carbohydrate diet) encountered trouble because he had inserted references to a pharmaceutical company and their product—safflower-oil capsules—safflower oil being one of the main features of the so-called Taller regimen. A federal court in Brooklyn convicted him of charges of conspiracy, postal fraud and food and drug violations, along with two of the executives of the publisher found to be in "cahoots" with Taller.

But this case was unusual. In general, authors, without benefit of facts, exercise their right to produce so-called health books. And you, in turn, should exercise your right to be selective, following the recommendations of established nutritional, dietetic, and medical groups, and passing over the nonsense which constantly comes our way from the health charlatans.

Diet faddists are just one of a group of health charlatans who will constantly be trying to sell you their counsel and products. If you are going to eat for good health, you'll have to be prepared to fight food faddism on all fronts. Chapter eight challenges some of our current versions of the age-old "art" of food faddism.

Chapter Eight

The Folly of Fads

Since earliest time, food faddists have been roaming around, masquerading as ministers of good health. Many eyeopening, entertaining books have been written about the subject of nutritional and medical quackery.

Having studied the subject, we have concluded that some small portion of the population has been and probably always will be victims of those who sell "magic cures", "natural foods", honey, vinegar, safflower oil capsules or even sea-water, and other substances as the magic keys to long life, perfect health and eternal youth.

Much of this nonsense is harmless up to a point, but nonsense, nonetheless.

We could not possibly list all the nostrums that are or have been in the "gyp parade" of the food charlatans. Many are here today and gone tomorrow; others change names and labels from one conviction to the next. But a few of them have been given a great deal of attention in recent years and it is worthwhile taking a close look at them and their advice.

Carlton Fredericks—"Foremost Nutritionist"

Perhaps the most influential advocate of vitamin and food therapy is Carlton Fredericks who claims on his book jackets to be "America's foremost nutritionist". He is now heard regularly on many U.S. radio stations.

According to a special supplement of *Nutrition Reviews* dealing with nutrition, misinformation and food faddism, he graduated from Alabama in 1931 with a major in English and a minor in political science; his only science courses comprised two hours of physiology and eight hours of elementary chemistry. He had miscellaneous jobs until about 1937, when he began to write advertising copy for the U.S. Vitamin Corporation and give sales talks, adopting the title "nutrition educator."

Nutrition Reviews states: "In 1945 Carlton Fredericks pleaded guilty to the illegal practice of medicine and paid a fine of $500." In 1955 he received his Ph.D. after coursework which included a thesis reported to be "in the area of nutrition." Actually, researchers who looked closely into this matter found that Fredericks took no course in nutrition at all, and his thesis was actually a study of communications and education, specifically a study of the female audience who listened to his radio programs!*

What type of advice does he give on his radio show?

Here are some examples of statements he has made to the public:

1. "Vitamin E should be included as a regular dietary supplement with all vitamin mixtures in view of the inadequate content of the average diet with respect to this vitamin."

2. "I can tell you the story too of a man who suffered with migraine headaches all his life until one day he took a multiple-vitamin supplement while he was in the middle of an attack. The headache disappeared."

3. "I recall too the story of a woman, a teacher, who came to a physician in tears, tears which had become quite common with her because her weeping was unprovoked. She said, 'I find myself crying in the classroom and startling the children,' and she said, 'I'm afraid they'll retire me medically before I get my pension.' She was given injections of the vitamin B-complex, and the weeping vanished as mysteriously as it had appeared."

On his show, Fredericks offers cures for cancer, heart disease, multiple sclerosis and poliomyelitis. He advocates the use of up to 100,000 units of vitamin A daily (for acne) and 150,000-200,000 for bronchial asthma. As we have pointed out earlier, such high doses of this fat-soluble vitamin can mean real trouble.

Additionally, you may hear this commentator informing you that

---

*From the article "Americans Love Hogwash" (page 6) by Edward H. Rynearson, M.D. in *Nutrition Reviews*, Supplement No. 1, July 1974.

vitamins and minerals can be used to treat a wide range of conditions including respiratory ailments, tooth decay, disturbed elimination, rheumatic fever, multiple sclerosis, lack of resistance to cancer, sexual frigidity and gray hair. But remember, these statements are made by a man who has no formal scientific, nutritional, health, or medical training.

Do we object to these exaggerated statements? Yes! And here's why:

1. Because of the false hopes they raise in those who think their aches and pains may disappear on taking the nutritional supplements recommended.

2. Because of the precious time that may be lost in seeking competent treatment for a serious disease.

3. Because of scanty savings that might better be used for food and shelter rather than vitamin and mineral preparations that will not be helpful in the condition for which they are recommended.

Unfortunately, our governmental regulatory agencies—particularly the Federal Communications Commission and the Food and Drug Administration—seldom take action against misinformation on health broadcast over the radio and TV. The best way for you to express your view is to write to the station and sponsors in your area and tell them that you think they have a responsibility to see that programs in the health field are not misleading and that they represent generally accepted views by those qualified by professional standards to express them.

Jerome Irving Rodale

The "guru of the organic cult" had as his claim to nutritional knowledge the fact that he was the son of a grocer.

He began his career as a federal tax auditor and moved on to become a manufacturer of electrical wiring accessories. Then in 1941 he learned about organic methods of gardening. And his new business career was set from then on.

Rodale maintained that we must eat "God's Way" in order to ensure long life. Specifically, we had to use only natural organic matter in fertilizing our soil, avoid eating anything that needed to be cooked, and eliminate wheat from the diet (it allegedly makes you "daffy"). Sugar and fluoridated water were other forbidden substances. His nutritional advice was promoted through his books (including *Organic Front* and *Happy People Rarely Get Cancer*) and the highly successful magazines and newsletters which regularly roll off the Rodale Press: *Prevention* (which tells us to "live it up and live longer," launched in 1950, now claiming an audience of over two million), *Organic Gardening and Farming* (begun in 1942, with a current circulation of about 700,000), and *Fitness for Living*.

Generally, the Rodale magazines are chock-full of charges against the FDA and food industry and occasionally one of us (F.J.S.) rates some unkind remark, all surrounded by pages and pages of advertisements for vitamin and mineral supplements.

It's hardly surprising to learn that with all his writings Rodale would be called both a genius and a crackpot. But which was he? We think you already know our answer, but read on anyway.

Rodale had no scientific training; his only formal background consisted of studying accounting at night school. Presumably this proved helpful, for as it turned out, he was basically a businessman. Yet he would make nutritional statements and offer advice as if he were qualified to do so.

He used to brag that he took seventy food-supplement tablets a day as "extra protection" against pollution and to "restore nutrients lost in the kitchen processing of food." Much of his advice was blatantly harmful; for instance, in one book, he claimed that the cure for prostatic disease was pumpkin seeds (to be eaten). How many men followed his advice, chose not to seek medical counsel for this serious ailment, and thus suffered the consequences is not known.

Mr. Rodale insisted that his healthy lifestyle would allow him to live to be 100 ("unless I'm run down by a sugar-crazed taxi driver"), but he didn't quite make it to the century mark. He died at the very respectable age of 73 while he and Dick Cavett were taping a show about the benefits of natural organic living.

Adelle Davis

Unlike many of the diet faddists who preceded and followed her, the late Adelle Davis did have a little professional background in the area of nutrition, even though it was obtained more than a generation ago.

She was trained in dietetics and nutrition at the University of California at Berkeley and received an M.S. in biochemistry from the University of Southern California Medical School in 1938. Her early contributions were scientific and her nutritional career showed promise. According to *Nutrition Reviews*, "Her former classmates and teachers are unanimous in their affectionate memories of her past promise and in their great distress about her present activities."

What foods did Adelle Davis recommend avoiding? At the top of her list were sugar, pasteurized or homogenized milk, white bread, food additives (of course) and unfertile eggs. For Ms. Davis, "proper diet" meant focusing on whole grains, fresh fruits and vegetables and at least two (fertile) eggs and a helping of cheese every day (she was not in agreement with the prevailing medical opinion linking foods high in saturated fats with heart disease).

Many of her books and articles contained serious medical errors. Edward H. Rynearson, M.D., emeritus professor of medicine at the Mayo Clinic and Mayo Foundation, read one of her best sellers, *Let's Get Well*, and found glaring examples of misquotations and inaccuracies. In chapter twelve, for example, of the fifty-seven references listed, twenty-seven instances had no data supporting her statement.

George Mann, M.D., Sc.D., of the Department of Biochemistry and Medicine at Vanderbilt University School of Medicine and a former member of Harvard's nutrition department, reviewed *Let's Eat Right to Keep Fit* and reported that the mistakes averaged one per page. Some of the errors were dangerous. One, for instance, was the suggestion that patients with nephrosis should take potassium chloride, a suggestion which according to medical experts is "extremely dangerous and even potentially lethal." Another was her implication that magnesium deficiency plays a major role in epilepsy and that magnesium alone is useful in the treatment of grand mal and petit mal. This statement is grossly misleading and therapeutically dangerous.

Much of her misleading advice has caused concern in the medical profession. For instance, when she took a stance against bottle-feeding and stated that crib deaths could be prevented by breast-feeding and diet supplements of vitamin E, at least one physician responded by sending a letter of complaint to the Federal Communications Commission asking for action against the statements. Ms. Davis replied to this physician's inquiry by writing, "Thank you so very much for correcting me. It was the first time I had heard that crib death occurs in infants while they are being breast fed. I am indeed sorry if words of mine have added to the suffering of parents whose infants have died." The problem with Ms. Davis' apologies is that they never got the attention her original inaccurate statements did.

At age sixty-nine, Adelle Davis was informed that she had bone cancer. She was initially shocked that, despite all her efforts to ensure healthful living, she could be affected by such a disease. But she advised her followers to continue to eat naturally.

Gaylord Hauser

A brief comment on a widely read individual who has been writing books—and reaping significant royalties—since the early 1950s. His primary "advice" revolves around the consumption of five "wonder foods"—skim milk, Brewer's yeast, wheat germ, yogurt and black-strap molasses. Eating a diet emphasizing these foods, he claimed, would add years to your life.

One of Hauser's latest books is *New Treasury of Secrets*, and it includes descriptions of "delicious wonder foods that quickly help to melt your fat—and conquer your craving to overeat," "the incredible Swiss apple diet that lowers blood pressure and reduces inches," "complete directions for growing your own precious vitamins," and information on "the super-energy eyeopener, drink it the minute you jump out of bed," and "how Gaylord Hauser saved the world's most glamourous women from mid-afternoon slump."

His books contain suggestions for making your own health foods. For instance, there is a German Egg Tonic he advises you concoct by mixing one fresh raw egg and a half a glass of sherry. It's best, he says, if you drink it with a straw.

A FATAL FORM OF FADDISM: LAETRILE

There are those who for years have been arguing that a substance known popularly as "laetrile" or more recently, as "vitamin B_{17}" is an effective means of preventing and curing cancer and therefore should be approved for use in this country. There is no evidence that laetrile is a useful cancer drug. But beyond that, its availability may actually cause deaths. William A. Nolan in his book, *A Doctor in Search of a Miracle* (Random House, 1974), tells the following story:

Dr. Nolan saw a patient he calls "Mary," a thirty-five-year-old married mother of three children. When Mary first came in to his office, Dr. Nolan diagnosed an early case of cancer of the uterus. He wanted to put her in the hospital right away and start treatment promptly. But he was unable to do so. As Mary's husband later told the story, she came home after hearing the diagnosis and immediately began to make plans to enter the hospital. But before she actually began undergoing medical treatment, Mary talked to a friend who spoke of another woman who supposedly had the same disease as Mary—cancer of the cervix. She had gone to Mexico for treatment, to a clinic just below the Texas border where they had given her a substance called laetrile. According to Mary's friend, this cleared everything right up, without radiation, surgery or anything else.

Mary insisted on trying this first. She was a sensible woman but the idea of either surgery or X-ray of her uterus frightened her, and she insisted on "giving the other method a try" before returning to Dr. Nolan. For awhile when she got back from Mexico, it did seem that she was getting better. The spotting symptoms that had caused her to seek medical treatment in the first place disappeared, and Mary—and even her husband—were convinced that the three thousand dollars they had spent for the "Mexico treatment" was worth it. Mary believed she was cured. It wasn't until six months had gone by and she was bleeding every day and losing strength fast that she became convinced that the laetrile was useless. She returned to Dr. Nolan's office, and he found that the cancer of the cervix had grown to the walls of the pelvis on both sides, had infiltrated the bladder from the front and the rectum from behind. There was no longer any effective treatment available. She died within a month.

Laetrile, or as properly named, amygdalin, is a cyanogenetic glycoside found in seeds of apricots, peaches and plums. Such glycosides are toxicants occurring naturally in foods. These substances have no food value or vitamin activity, although, as mentioned, the misnomer vitamin B_{17} is used in the promotion of laetrile.

The use of laetrile to treat cancer was originally proposed by Ernst Krebs, M.D., who believed that the substance would be broken down by an enzyme in cancerous tissues to liberate cyanide which would "kill the cancer." When this explanation was proved false, others were offered in support of an application to the FDA for approval of laetrile as a drug. Such applications have been rejected because of insufficient scientific evidence that the product was safe and effective in the treatment of cancer. As of this writing, laetrile is being approved by a number of state legislators despite the widely accepted conclusion that it is ineffective and, as was demonstrated in the case of "Mary," downright dangerous.

FIGHT FOOD MYTHS WITH NUTRITIONAL REALITY

We could list many more food faddists of the past and present. But we won't. Instead, consider a few of the food myths—and then the realities—which you may read about in books, newspapers and magazines.

Myth: Organically grown foods are more nutritious than "chemically fertilized foods."
Reality: Organically grown foods are identical in nutritional quality to those grown by more conventional means.

The owners of some health-food stores may lead you to believe otherwise. But repeated reputable scientific studies conclude that the two varieties are indistinguishable.

Generally speaking, organically grown foods boast of two unique qualities: growth without benefit of chemical fertilizers and freedom from any type of pesticides and their residues. The consumer advantages to be derived from these two differences are questionable while the disadvantages have recently become clear.

Those who have "gone organic" maintain that "natural fertilizers," unlike their commercial counterparts, are full of the type of rich vitamins and minerals on which plants thrive. But all fertilizers, whether they are commercially processed or derived from living organisms, must be broken down to inorganic compounds of nitrogen, potassium and phosphorus before the plants can use them. Only carbon dioxide can be used directly by a plant. When the fertilizer is transformed into the type of nutrients which will promote growth, even the most discerning plant cannot identify its origin.

So fertilizers, organic or otherwise, cannot yield improved nutritional quality. You can't increase the vitamin content of a food by altering the way it is grown. Its vitamin content is largely genetically determined. But obviously fertilization effects crop yield!

There is evidence that organic fertilizers may also pose a health risk. First, it has been shown that fertilizers of animal origin can be lacking in the type of nutrients necessary for ideal farming conditions. Processed fertilizers, on the other hand, can be more consistent in quality and can correct for deficiencies that may exist in the soil.

Second, there is evidence that the use of animal or human manure may be dangerous. According to our former colleague Dr. Jean Mayer, ". . . biologically speaking, [organic foods] tend to become the most contaminated, as all organic fertilizers of animal or human origin are obviously the most likely to contain gastrointestinal parasites."

Dr. Mayer's statement is reinforced by recent reports from South Korea and Holland where human sewage was being used to fertilize crops, that significant portions of the population suffered from roundworms, hookworm and other parasites. Of course not all organically grown foods present these types of problems. It is only when the organically derived fertilizer is not used properly that an incomplete chemical breakdown occurs, and disease becomes a possibility. With commercially processed fertilizer, however, a risk of this nature is never present.

Don't be taken in by the organic food myths. If you find specialty foods at your health-food outlet—foods you can't find elsewhere and foods you like—by all means buy them and enjoy them. But don't go to health-food-land expecting to buy foods with unique health-promoting qualities. You'll find those kinds of food at any supermarket—at a significantly lower price!

Myth: Lecithin is nature's protection against heart attacks.
Reality: There is no evidence that lecithin protects against heart attacks or any other disease.

Lecithin is a natural emulsifying agent. It has been used for many years as a food additive in mayonnaise, salad dressings, and chocolate to maintain the stability of the oil ingredients.

But it's not a key to preventing heart attacks. Some food faddists contend that lecithin can cure arthritis, high blood pressure and gallbladder problems, while also improving brain power. Others recommend it in conjunction with cider vinegar, kelp and vitamin B_6 as a weight-reduction method. Sorry, it doesn't work.

The theory linking heart disease prevention and lecithin consumption is that the substance can disperse cholesterol in the blood so that it will not become attached to the artery walls. Indeed, faddist

Gaylord Hauser, in his *New Treasury of Secrets*, says that while eggs are high in cholesterol, the lecithin in them keeps "cholesterol on the move." Nonsense!

The body manufactures its own lecithin, and there is no medical evidence to suggest that we need additional amounts of it. Heart specialists have expressed concern that those who are buying lecithin tablets, chewable wafers and oil solutions are deluding themselves—continuing to smoke, omitting exercise and proper diet—that is, not giving attention to the variables which have been linked with higher probabilities of heart disease.

There is no evidence at this point that excessive doses of lecithin actually do any harm—except perhaps to your limited food budget.

Myth: Some foods, honey for example, have "magical" properties.
Reality: The claims of honey and other "wonder foods" have no scientific basis.

Eating habits are very susceptible to rumor. Throughout history, someone would publicly acclaim the wonders of a specific food and gullible listeners would eagerly try it.

Probably the leading miracle food of the day is honey. One obviously enthusiastic health-food store owner said, "I recommended it [honey] for ulcers, cancers and mostly for healthy people as a prevention of both." Others who have concluded that there is money in honey claim that their product does truly miraculous things—for instance, causing chickens to lay more eggs and ensuring the return of fertility in post-menopausal-age women.

Sorry, honey tastes good. But that's about it. And it doesn't suddenly acquire magic potential, not even when you mix it with vinegar (as some faddists might lead you to believe).

Myth: Teflon cooking utensils are dangerous, and aluminum foil contains chemicals which are released by oven heat.
Reality: Teflon cookware is perfectly safe, and so is aluminum foil.

All materials that are put on the market to be used in the cooking or storage of food are safe. Only those who are trying to sell a competing product will try to convince you otherwise!

Myth: Frequently, weariness and exhaustion during the day is a sign of hypoglycemia ("low blood sugar").
Reality: Hypoglycemia occurs very rarely and only in most unusual cases is it the explanation for feelings of fatigue.

Recent publicity in the United States' popular press has led many consumers to believe that the occurrence of hypoglycemia is widespread in this country and is the cause of depression, allergies, nervous breakdowns, alcoholism, juvenile delinquency and, among other things, inadequate sexual performance. It is not. Because of the possible misunderstanding about this matter, three organizations of physicians and scientists (the American Diabetes Association, the Endocrine Society and the American Medical Association) have issued the following statement for the public. Read it and remember it so you can respond when your local faddist starts talking about low blood sugar and how to handle it!

> Hypoglycemia means a low level of blood sugar. When it occurs, it is often attended by symptoms of sweating, shakiness, trembling, anxiety, fast heart action, headache, hunger sensations, brief feelings of weakness and occasionally seizures and coma. However, the majority of people with these kinds of symptoms do not have hypoglycemia; a great many patients with anxiety reactions present with similar symptoms.

Carlton Fredericks, among others, will try to convince you that some 20 million Americans are suffering from this disease, and that low blood sugar is the underlying cause of many ills. But such statements have no basis in fact. But like many fallacious beliefs, the belief in hypoglycemia has engendered a form of treatment— generally requiring a steady stream of office visits at $25 or more each.

FOR SALE: COMMON SENSE

Common sense is a hard product to sell.
Why is it so much easier for pseudo-scientists to sell food fads than it is for ethical scientists with years of the best training available and backed by federal, state, industrial, and university laboratories to convince people of the completely good nutrition that is easily obtainable in our ordinary foods?
Every qualified nutritionist who speaks or writes on common-

sense nutrition gets letters from a belligerent group of people who insist that to be nutritious, wheat mustn't be grown with manu-factured fertilizer, that vegetables mustn't be canned or frozen, that milk mustn't be pasteurized, that water mustn't be fluoridated, that honey and brown sugar are more nutritious than white sugar, and a dozen variations on these themes.

Let the food faddists and so-called health-food stores guarantee what they call the "curative properties" of such things as honey and vinegar, organically grown vegetables, stone ground flour, sunflower seeds, kelp, sea salt, and the trace minerals in the many odd com-binations they so readily put together with added vitamins. We can't do it because we scientists use only information proved by scientific testing, and with adequate controls, to be true—not the testimonials that are so often the support of the faddists.

It has been proved that chemical fertilizers greatly increase crop yield and do not harm or lessen nutritive value. It has been proved that there is no difference between synthetic vitamins and natural ones. It has been proved over and over again that fluoridation of community water supplies will result in a 50- to 70-percent reduction in dental decay, not its elimination, and that it is safe, safe, safe—for all ages and in any state of health.

We are false to ourselves, and to every advance science has made, if we allow a vocal letter-writing minority to scare us into buying special foods or products advertised as cure-alls or into denying our children the benefits of fluoridated water. Unfortunately, this letter-writing minority has had increasing influence with many of our politicians who do not have the courage to stand up to them—votes!

And what happens when a gullible customer finds that a "perfect food" does not change his health or his weight? Does he return to eating a common-sense variety of foods or does he cast about for another product touted to be a panacea for everything from bad tem-per to obesity?

It is so simple to achieve good nutrition these days. Our stores are crowded with the best food that has ever been available—made so by the same precise, time-consuming, scientific processes that have given us other advances that assure us the good American life.

Why should we allow food faddists to keep us from enjoying the products of good, modern nutrition? Would you let anyone send you back to the days of no automobiles or no washing machines?

Of course not! We Americans pride ourselves on taking advantage of every available technological advance and want the rest of the world to share the best with us.

So let us accept, enjoy, and profit from the products of our food scientists and relegate food faddism and its horse-and-buggy, scrub-board ideas to the dark past. This is hard to do. Food faddism and quackery are just too profitable and the penalties too light for the few who get caught. More and more people are getting into the game every day. What is needed are a few jail sentences that are not sus-pended and some fines comparable with the profits.

HOW TO SPOT A QUACK*

Following is an informative list of check points published some years ago by the American Medical Association. The various organi-zations in our country dedicated to the health and well-being of our people are gravely concerned about the problem of food and medical faddism and quackery.

The reasons for this concern are chiefly two:

1. A person who is taken in by silver-tongued purveyors of misinformation stands a very good chance of endangering his own health as well as that of his family. Except for eating too much, Americans in this day and age have to go out of their way, nutritionally speaking, to become poorly nourished. Food faddism is one sure way! Also, putting one's faith in the cura-tive powers of some "magic" food or formula can lead to neglect of a real disorder.

2. The fantastic drain on the family pocketbook is one of the hazards of food quackery. It has been estimated that the American public spends two billion dollars each year on gim-micks, reducing pills, misleading books, diet plans, "organic" foods, fancy machines and devices. This makes the "medicine man" of the carnival days look like a piker.

In general there are two types of food quacks. There is the in-dividual food faddist who sincerely believes in the bizarre and miraculous qualities of one specific food or a combination of foods.

---

*For further information on this subject, we heartily recommend that you read *The Health Robbers* edited by Stephen Barrett, M.D., and Gilda Knight, foreword by Ann Landers, published in 1976 by the George F. Stickley Co.

He is also a great "converter." This person is relatively harmless—just misguided.

The real villain is the quack or faddist who spreads his misinformation for personal profit. Actually, the charlatan himself need not be a faddist; he just thrives on the gullible. You need to be able to spot these people.

1. They *always* have something to sell: a course of lectures, pills, nature foods, tonics, food supplements, diet plans, rollers (to roll off the fat), books, even pots and pans.

2. They guarantee quick cures—on a money-back basis, "if your arthritis isn't cured in eight days."

3. They often claim to be "medical experts" or "nutritionists" with some secret formula or knowledge that will cure, and they usually boast about membership in a "scientific society" with a high-sounding name.

4. They use testimonials and case histories to prove that their product is miraculous, not facts based on carefully controlled studies, published in reputable medical journals and confirmed by independent workers.

5. They distort scientific data to suit their own ends.

6. They say that what you are doing now is deadly—the food you are eating is poisoned, the way you cook it is all wrong.

7. They claim to be persecuted by medical men or governmental agencies, because, they insist, the medical profession and the Food and Drug Administration are corrupt and influenced by big business.

Remember, the faddist and quack isn't interested in you—just your bank account.

Chapter Nine
"Dietary Goals for the United States": A Critique

In early 1977, the United States Printing Office released a report prepared by the staff of the Select Committee on Nutrition and Human Needs of the United States Senate. Technically known by the title "Dietary Goals for the United States," the document was generally referred to as "The McGovern Report," after Senator George McGovern, chairman of the committee.

Specifically, the report recommended six goals:

1. Increase carbohydrate consumption to account for 55-60 percent of the energy (caloric) intake.

2. Reduce overall fat consumption from approximately 40 to 30 percent of energy intake.

3. Reduce saturated fat consumption to account for about 10 percent of total energy intake; and balance that with poly-unsaturated and monounsaturated fats, which should account for about 10 percent of energy intake each.

4. Reduce cholesterol consumption to about 300 mg a day.

5. Reduce sugar consumption by about 40 percent to account for 15 percent of total energy intake.

6. Reduce salt consumption by about 50 to 85 percent to approximately 3 grams a day.

Obviously, from what we've said throughout this book, there are points in these goals which we heartily endorse. But there are others which we question, particularly the goal related to sugar.

Here we present some general comments on the so-called "McGovern Report."

"Dietary Goals"

Americans today are vitally interested in the subject of nutrition. Each year they buy hundreds of thousands of books which offer diets promising to "save your life" or reduce unwanted pounds. Almost all popular magazines and major newspaper syndicates carry regular features on nutrition and health. National radio and television programs focus on food, diet and nutrition and their relationship to physical and mental well-being.

But although the interest is there, it is not always easy for American eaters to distinguish food facts from food fallacies. Nutritional nonsense now surrounds us, and only the most discerning consumer can choose wisely from the plethora of advice which is offered both by professionally trained nutritionists and medical scientists—and self-appointed "experts" whose only apparent "credential" in the food area is that they eat three times a day.

It is therefore commendable that the United States Senate formed a Committee on Nutrition and Human Needs to sift through facts, figures and opinions in the areas of nutrition and health with a view to setting forth guidelines aimed at improving the nutritional and general health status of Americans. Ideally, such a committee would serve the function of moderator in assessing the state of knowledge in the field and in interpreting areas of conflicts and controversy. The final report of such an effort would then be (a) a summary of current scientific knowledge about specific aspects of nutrition and health; (b) an acknowledgment of legitimate areas of scientific disagreement, but presentation of the "drift" which the majority of scientific evidence takes; (c) a statement which clearly distinguishes between established facts, apparent associations, and purely hypothetical links between diet and disease; and (d) a formulation of general dietary goals, making recommendations for diet modification where there is a clear consensus of medical scientific evidence to support such recommendations.

Unfortunately, the committee report "Dietary Goals for the United States" accomplished none of the desirable ends.

First, instead of offering a balanced presentation of what is often a controversial and highly emotionally-charged subject, the report reflects the views of a small group of vocal, opinionated and even nonprofessional individuals, in many cases overlooking the consensus of the medical scientific community, as reflected in the professional literature. Second, those preparing "Dietary Goals" appear to be unable or unwilling to distinguish between established relationships of nutrition and health and hypothetical relationships which have either been rejected by the majority of those conducting scientific inquiries or are merely in the preliminary hypothesis-formation stage, the focus of new research endeavors. Third, while some of the six recommendations do have sound, solid, epidemiological and clinical bases, others are derived from assumptions grounded only in speculation. Here the four primary flaws of the report may be summarized:

1. "Dietary Goals for the United States" inaccurately includes sugar, on the same list as fats, saturated fats, cholesterol, alcohol and salt, as a dietary factor responsible for death-dealing diseases. There is no known scientific reason for including sugar on such a list.

2. The report frequently states as established fact observations which at best can be described as rumor or speculation.

3. The committee displays a willingness—indeed, eagerness— to recommend drastic dietary change without benefit of evidence, apparently based on an underlying assumption that our diet was more health-promoting earlier in this century than it is now; that our food preparation and distribution systems are unnecessarily complex and that we could benefit physically and psychologically from more "natural" living; and that although evidence for the desirablitiy of certain dietary modifications may be lacking, "it wouldn't hurt" to return to the early twentieth-century eating pattern.

4. The report frequently overlooks realities, namely that eating is more than a biological experience and is indeed a pleasure of life. A difficult-to-define, but noticeable characteristic of the report is the underlying philosophy that what we enjoy (sugar and sugar-containing products, for example) may for that reason alone be harmful, that eating should be a function solely aimed at meeting a daily list of recommended nutrients, that food-for-fun is somehow bad.

The report of the Senate Select Committee is a serious source of concern for a number of reasons.

First, any formal government statement about something of such high priority interest as nutrition and health will be taken very seriously by the unscientifically-oriented public. Indeed this should be the case. But this is also an imperative reason that such reports be accurate, not opinionated, rambling and out of step with scientific knowledge. Second, adherence to the goals presented in the report may interfere with medical investigations into the actual causes of killer diseases. For example, a preoccupation with sugar as a cause of diabetes (a concern which has no scientific basis but is emphasized in the report) will only serve to distract research efforts in this area, delaying the further identification of real risk factors in this disease. Third, issuance of governmental statements based on hypothesis and opinion rather than firm scientific fact only leads to questions about the credibility of public health policy in general. Perhaps, an uninformed consumer may conclude, the health hazards of cigarette smoking are as flimsy as those on sugar. Fourth, the report sets a dangerous precedent in suggesting in a number of the specific goals and related recommendations relatively drastic action based on tenuous evidence instead of maintaining strenuous defini- tions for the identification of disease risk factors and, where these strenuous definitions are not met, presenting the full range of avail- able facts and letting the consumer decide for himself what the recommended course of action should be.

GENERAL COMMENTS ON THE SHORTCOMINGS AND LIMITATIONS OF "DIETARY GOALS"

1. There is an obvious built-in bias of the report which commun- icates even to the most casual reader that modern food-processing techniques, the use of food additives and pesticides are inherently either bad or unnecessary and that a return to a more "natural" life would in itself be desirable. This general philosophy sets the pattern for the report's presentation although there is never any solid evidence to back up these premises.

2. There is a willingness on the part of the committee's staff to accept simplistic statements which have no basis in fact. For ex- ample, in a section on obesity it is stated that "the water content

and bulk in fruits and vegetables and bulk of whole grain can bring satisfaction of appetite more quickly than can foods high in fat and sugar." To our knowledge, there is no scientific evidence to back up such a contention. Indeed, just the opposite might be argued: for many individuals "appetite" has a large psychological component which cannot be satisfied without some fat and sugar. Additionally, while a high-in-fiber or high-in-vegetable diet may temporarily appease one's appetite, it may well not have the same long-term satiety value of a diet which does include some fat and sugar.

3. The committee appeared willing to make recommendations on the basis of a lack of knowledge as opposed to direct information. For example, the staff notes that our knowledge about the need of the human body for various trace elements and "micronutrients" is not complete. On the basis of this lack of information the recommendation is made to increase consumption of fruits, vegetables and whole grains just in case we might improve our status with regard to these nutrients.

This is an unscientific basis for making such an encompassing recommendation when there is *no* basis that we have any type of ill health due to a lack of micronutrients that might be remedied by these foods. Meats also have micronutrients!

4. Statements are made in somewhat ominous tones without any indication of what the basis for concern is. In his introduction, Senator McGovern notes that "last year every man, woman and child in the United States consumed 125 pounds of fat, and 100 pounds of sugar . . . that's a formidable quantity of fat and sugar." The obvious questions are: Were these quantities actually eaten and what is the evidence for this? Who established that these were "formidable quantities"? Why does a statement of pound intake over a period of a year of a specific category of nutrient necessarily implicate it as a hazard?

5. The entire report has a negative orientation. One might conclude after reading "Dietary Goals" that the United States had the most dismal health, nutrition and food record in the world, whereas we probably have the best. Certainly a national statement of nutrition guidelines should make some note of the nutritional successes this country has had, noting that in the past seventy-five years our country has developed a plentiful supply of foods, providing a growing population, and much of the rest of the world, with a variety of nutritious, safe, attractive, and relatively inexpensive diets on a year-

round basis. The most recent nationwide surveys on nutritional status (the Health and Nutrition Examination Surveys of the U.S. Population Ages 1-74, taken in 1971-1972) indicated that for the most part all age groups (for all races and income levels) had adequate amounts of protein, calcium, vitamin A and vitamin C. The major dietary deficiency at all age levels was in iron intake.

The contributions made in the area of public health and nutrition have had a marked effect on life expectancy. (For instance, a white male born between 1900 and 1902 could, at the time of birth, expect to live only forty-eight years. Today the life expectancy for males at birth is somewhat over seventy years—and for women seventy-four or more. Additionally, changes in food production and distribution have had a dramatic impact on the time spent in food production and preparation and the "processed foods" much maligned in "Dietary Goals" have made life easier and more enjoyable for millions of American men and women.

6. There is frequent use of the words "may be," "could be," "might possibly" in the report. Pure speculation does not merit a place in Senate committee guidelines. The fact that those words are used—and reference is made to alleged health hazards of specific foods and food additives without the benefit of evidence—confirms the presence of an underlying preconceived philosophy about what is and is not right for the American diet. One wonders how many of the nonprofessional staff might have been "natural food enthusiasts."

7. The somewhat dictatorial, often supercilious, approach to dietary recommendations is disturbing. For example, after indicting sugar as a "nutrient danger" and cause of diabetes and tooth decay, the committee goes on to refer to a "total elimination of soft drinks from the diet." Perhaps committee members should have taken note of the reality that Americans like and enjoy soft drinks and have no intention of following a "total elimination" pattern.

8. The report is often naive in the sense that it overlooks obvious factors which explain increased demand of certain foods and beverages. In discussing (and, by implication, deploring) the shift in carbohydrate consumption and decline in use of starches, the staff writers note that "a key factor may be the rise in real income, permitting a movement away from diets high in greens, beans and whole grains, which had been enforced by economics." It should have been clear to the committee that when consumers had the option (made possible by greater availability and disposable income), they *by*

choice reduced what the committee refers to as "complex carbohydrates." This shift away from starch, then, was not necessarily foisted upon consumers by the food industry. More likely, the sequence was just the opposite: because of the perceived consumer desirability of products containing sugar and fats over greens, beans and whole grains, industry responded by making products more available. Consumers here, then, are not victims but rather initiators of the change.

9. The section discussing the sociocultural implications of diet can only be described as "elitist." The statement to the effect that "an increasingly mechanized approach to the provision of food may have not only potential for negative nutritional effect but also a negative psychological effect" has no place in a factual presentation of nutrition knowledge. Diet selection and taste are very personally determined, and there is no one "superior" way of meeting nutritional needs as long as moderation, balance and variety are considered.

10. With the impressive number of citations available in the medical-scientific literature, it was puzzling to note the heavy reliance of the report on sources such as *The New York Times* and the *Washington Post*, hardly scientific sources.

11. Inclusion of anecdotal material (e.g., citing a study based on twelve individuals of an alleged relationship of migraine headache and use of salt; and using as a source a "letter to the editor" of a medical journal condemning MSG) when there is extensive literature on the subject is inexcusable in a report which purports to be thorough and unbiased.

12. The report makes reference to irrelevant material. For instance, in the section dealing with sugar it was stated (correctly) that there is "no clear link" between sugar consumption and risk of heart disease. The question is: why was it mentioned at all? There is no clear link between sugar consumption and the frequency of automobile accidents either, but that was not mentioned. The implication is that "maybe after all there is something here, it's just that it has not been proven yet."

Additionally, and along the same lines, it was irrelevant when discussing the "total elimination of soft drinks" to insert statements suggesting caffeine isn't good for us either. The subject matter at hand was sugar, not caffeine. But even here the report refers to an article in *Medical World News* (not a scientific publication) that "suspected connections between caffeine and [several diseases] have been investigated but that evidence is not strong enough to cause caffeine to be adjudged a risk factor in these diseases." Then why even mention it except for gaining a little publicity? Too many people read only what they want to read, remember what they want to remember, and that appears to be the case with those who prepared this report.

13. In a number of areas, there was a tendency to confuse priorities which might be recommended or required for one small portion of the population with those that are applicable to only one small segment. For example, in stressing the desirability for more complex carbohydrates in the diet, a major reason offered fell under the subtitle "diabetes," indicating that a high complex carbohydrate diet is important in the treatment of diabetics because it reduces the threat of atherosclerosis and hyperlipidemia. That may or may not be so, but regardless, it is not a relevant observation for general dietary goals for U.S. citizens.

14. A basic theme of the committee report is that things have changed—and change is bad. There is great emphasis on the fact that there has been a shift in proportional consumption of carbohydrates —in favor of sugars, away from starches. What was never made clear in the report was the common sense observation that change or, specifically, increased use is not inherently bad.

15. There were a number of blatant errors in the report. Under Goal #2, "One of the principal reasons for reducing the consumption of fat is to make a place in the diet for complex carbohydrates which generally carry higher levels of micro-nutrients than fat without the complications of fat." As far as we know, this is *not* one of the principal reasons for this recommendation. Indeed it is the reduction of fat, particularly saturated fat, per se which is considered beneficial to health, not an increase in micronutrients.

Additionally, it was stated that "fat and sugar are relatively low in vitamins and minerals." This statement is incorrect. Except for vitamin A in some fats, fats and sugars are free from vitamins and minerals.

Furthermore, it is stated "only foods of animal origin have significant amounts of cholesterol." The correct statement is "only foods of animal origin have any cholesterol."

16. In a number of areas, the report simplified to the point where it is in error. For instance, in quoting Dr. George Briggs, professor of nutrition at the University of California, stating that improved nutri-

tion might cut the nation's health bill by one-third, the committee overlooks the obvious fact that a reduction of some of the chronic diseases discussed in the report may indeed lead to a higher national health bill in that, if the committee's premises are correct, people would live longer and older people are in need of more medical services. Further, while Dr. Briggs is knowledgeable in nutrition, particularly the nutrition of chickens, he is not an authority on the economics of human health.

Obesity is indeed an important American nutritional problem but the report gives scant attention to it. And the attention to it certainly should not be included under the heading of one particular class of nutrients, that is, fats. Obesity represents a positive balance of calories—an excess of caloric intake over caloric expenditure. The excess can come from starch, sugar, protein, fats or alcohol, taken with or between meals. Additionally, obesity can also result from inadequate caloric expenditure without an increased caloric intake ... or it may be the combination of eating too much and not getting enough exercise. But to simplify this complex problem by attributing it to excess fat intake is erroneous and misleading. Alcoholic beverages are an increasing source of calories to many Americans, yet this is not even mentioned in the report.

Along the same lines, it is stated that "an increased consumption of complex carbohydrates is likely to ease the problem of weight control." There is no basis for such a statement. Obesity is the result of excessive intake of calories, whether those calories are from meat or from "complex carbohydrates" such as those in spaghetti, rice or cereal.

17. Many of the theoretical statements made throughout the report overlook the reality of living in a modern world with an expanding population. It may be fine to praise farm fresh produce, but urban dwellers are faced with a practical problem of meeting nutrient needs on a year-round basis.

Further, emphasizing the nutritional superiority of brown rice overlooks the difference in shelf life between brown and processed rice and the propensity of brown rice for rancidity; it also reminds us of the nutritional nonsense (and real hazard) of the Zen Macrobiotic Diet which favors brown rice. Statements about vitamin and mineral loss in canned vegetables neglect to note that the losses are relatively slight and have no practical implication, given the fact that most Americans receive B vitamins and other nutrients from a wide variety of sources and receive more than they physiologically need anyway. Comparing the fat content of potato chips with "natural potatoes" neglects to point out that most people eating mashed or baked potatoes do add some type of margarine or butter to it. Contrary to what the report indicates, ten medium potato chips and one cup of mashed potatoes with milk and margarine each contain the same amount of fat (eight grams). American and French fried potatoes are "natural potatoes" and not devoid of fat!

18. The report contains many statements long on opinion and short on facts. In the discussion of food additives, reference is made to "continuing discoveries of apparent connections between certain types of additives and cancer." This statement is incorrect. There has *never* been any published scientific account linking the use of any food additives with human cancer, nor is there any degree of evidence from animal experiments which even suggests that additives pose risks as human carcinogens. The report refers to an alleged relationship of food additive ingestion (particularly colorings and flavorings) and hyperkinesis, or hyperactivity in children. Again, there is no evidence that this realtionship is valid. Indeed the alleged link of additives and behavioral problems is the opinion of one West Coast allergist, and reviews by a series of professionals from the fields of pediatrics, nutrition, psychiatry and other areas find no basis for his conclusion.

Despite the lack of information, the above two observations were used to justify the conclusion that Americans should "reduce additive consumption to the greatest degree possible." Such a conclusion is very unfortunate as it only serves to further intensify the anxieties of Americans who are already suffering from "chemical phobia" and a poor understanding of the term "cancer-causing agent."

CONCLUSION ON THE McGOVERN REPORT ON DIETARY GOALS FOR THE U.S.

We find the report deficient in many respects, primarily because it is a political report prepared by a non-professional staff who, in our opinion, had pretty fixed ideas on what was to be in the report even before any hearings were held. The report is not scientific, though it comes from a Senate committee and is supported (in part) by three and one-half pages of references (many of which are pseudo-scientific).

It is true that the nonprofessional staff received help in the drafting of the final report from an excellent experimental nutritionist; however, the help was too little and too late to be of much help. The committee and the staff did not avail themselves of the abundance of medical-nutritional help from professional organizations such as the American Heart Association, American Diabetes Association, Food and Nutrition Board, GRAS Committee of the Federation of American Biological Societies, or National Nutrition Consortium.

The report is weak in dealing with two of the major nutrition problems of this country, obesity and tooth decay. Not a word in the report refers to the growing contribution that alcoholic beverages make to the caloric intake of many Americans. The role of physical activity as an important factor in the avoidance and treatment of obesity is barely mentioned. The role of the mineral nutrient, fluoride, and the fluoridation of community water supplies as the only realistic way to reduce by more than half the incidence of tooth decay is not even mentioned. No mention is made of the importance of reducing food waste.

While a footnote points out that estimates of food supplies are based on "disappearance data" and not on actual food ingested, nevertheless, the report implies that the various comments and recommendations relate to foods actually consumed.

To end this critical review on a positive note, the report has brought the subject of nutrition to the attention of the Congress and the public, and perhaps as a result more realistic dietary goals for the United States will eventually result.

* * * * *

Since this chapter was set in type, a second edition of Dietary Goals was released. It was good to see the emphasis that nutrition should become a "major consideration of . . . agricultural policy". With the "McGovern Committee" abolished on December 31, 1977 and nutrition added to the Senate Agriculture Committee this might be possible. The second edition rightly gives increased emphasis to the avoidance of obesity, contains a specific footnote on alcohol consumption, and makes minor changes in the original suggestions relative to consumption of sugar, meats, and salt. However, most of our criticism of the original report still applies to the second edition. Senator Percy in a minority statement commented "I have serious reservations about certain aspects of the report." And so do we!

Chapter Ten
Eating for Good Health: An Overview

If you have completed the previous nine chapters of this book, we hope you have reached the conclusion that the best diet for you and your health is one that provides the physiologic and psychologic values from food that will permit you to obtain and maintain the best health permitted by your genetic potential.

As we conclude, we will take the opportunity to summarize the most important guidelines for eating for good health.

Daily Food Guides

The food one eats is a very personal matter. Normally, most people resist eating a diet outlined completely and specifically by someone else. The comments and complaints about food that are so common in college dormitories and other institutionalized settings illustrate the emotional and personal value people place upon selecting their own foods. Menus planned for groups of people may be nutritionally adequate in every way, and yet these menus may fail to allow for the fact that one or more or the foods included may not be eaten for cultural or personal reasons. Planned but uneaten food serves no nutritional purpose in a diet! Clearly then, it is necessary to provide a complete easy-to-use guide for the individual to use in planning his daily food intake. The merits of good nutrition are gaining ever-increasing recognition, but it is the application of this knowledge to daily living that must be achieved.

The "Basic Four," which we discussed at length in chapter three, is a simple concept for planning adequate nutrition on a daily basis to outline the variety of foods that will provide a "balanced diet" that includes the essential nutrients. Although not structured to enumerate all foods needed daily, it does provide a very practical framework for meal planning. Sugar or refined fats and oils are not included because these substances, although they are important in nutrition, mainly provide calories and are usually not lacking in American diets.

The foods groups mentioned in the Basic Four are:

1. Meat, poultry, fish, and other excellent protein sources;
2. Milk and its products;
3. Vegetables and fruits;
4. Cereals and their products.

For practical purposes of food selection, the average adult can very simply meet his recommended dietary allowance by consuming daily two servings from the milk group, five ounces from the meat group, four servings from the bread group, and four from the vegetable-fruit group.

Meat Group

This contains meats, poultry, fish, and legumes such as dried beans, peas and nuts. All are good sources of protein. In addition, they supply vitamins of the B complex such as thiamine, riboflavin, niacin, B_6 and B_{12}, and the mineral iron.

Meat also brings calories, fat and cholesterol to the diet, the former in rather large amounts. For example, an average serving of roast beef (3½ ounces) may contain 350 Calories, an ounce of fat (even "lean" meat contains 5 to 10 percent fat), and 70 milligrams of cholesterol. The businessman who sits down to a one-pound steak is facing 1440 Calories (half his total daily need), 4 to 5 ounces of fat, and 320 milligrams of cholesterol (300 is the top daily limit recommended by the American Heart Association) from just one steak alone!

Milk Group

Milk and milk products supply more calcium and phosphorus per serving than any other food. It is difficult to meet the recommendations for calcium without the use of milk or cheese. In addition, milk provides valuable sources of protein, many of the B vitamins (especially riboflavin), vitamin A (if the milk is whole milk), and vitamin D if it has been added to the milk as it should be. Users of skim milk, dry skim milk powder, or low-fat milk should choose those labeled as having vitamin A and D added. The original vitamins have been removed along with the fat in these types of milk.

Adults and weight-conscious girls seem particularly prone to omit milk from the daily eating pattern. The new low-fat milks, with fewer calories and less cholesterol, or fat-free skim milk is a good solution.

Fruit and Vegetable Group

This is one of the most interesting yet most neglected of the food groups. It is the source of some 90 percent of vitamin C, at least 60 percent of vitamin A, and much of the fiber in the average diet.

Dietary surveys indicate that C is the vitamin most often found in less than recommended amounts in diets of all age groups. Vitamin A often is in short supply in diets of the elderly.

How easily these shortages could be corrected! One serving of a vitamin-C-rich food daily and one serving of a vitamin-A-rich food at least every other day are sufficient for almost everyone. Two or three additional servings of vegetables or fruit complete the daily suggested quantities of fruit and vegetables.

In addition to vitamins A and C, fruits and vegetables provide important amounts of minerals, folic acid, fiber (bulk) and carbohydrate. They also add texture, color and variety—important psychologic values of any diet.

Bread and Cereal Group

Bread and cereal are often misunderstood and inaccurately described as being fattening, overprocessed, almost worthless, and full of air and additives. Far from the truth! Bread and cereal are valuable sources of carbohydrate, protein, thiamine, riboflavin, niacin and iron. In fact, it is difficult to obtain a sufficient quantity of thiamine and iron if this group is excluded from diet.

In the quibble for calories, it scarcely seems logical to avoid eating bread at sixty-five or seventy Calories per slice and then eat extra meat at seventy-five to ninety Calories per ounce. But, of course, no single food is fattening; body fat is accumulated only when total caloric intake exceeds caloric expenditure.

Despite recent concerns about overprocessing, white bread outsells whole-grain breads by roughly five to one. Because the American taste prefers white bread, enrichment laws have been enacted in about half the states; in the others it is done voluntarily. Enrichment requires that the important vitamins and minerals—thiamine, riboflavin, niacin and iron—which are partially removed when flour is milled, are replaced to a level equivalent to those in whole-wheat flour or bread.

Other Foods

Few of us eat without including a myriad of fats, sugars, spreads, dressing and "complements" to our foods. Think of all those desserts, beverages and snacks! Indeed, these additions may increase the caloric value of daily foods by 25 percent or more.

Let us put the foods we eat into perspective. When the need arises to cut calorie intake, the "other foods" should be sacrificed. The foods from the four Basic Food Groups should be left intact.

Food "Chemicals"

As we elaborated upon in our book *Panic in the Pantry* (and here in chapter five), there is no need to panic in the pantry. Before being caught up in the current wave of chemical phobia that is going around, remember that ALL foods, indeed all things, are made of chemicals. With the additive scare which has gripped Americans in the past five years, one might believe that only artificial products were full of strange-sounding concoctions.

Natural foods are not necessarily better.

You will continue to read and hear stories about how additives are dangerous, have not been tested, and are put in our foods so companies can make more money. The reality is, however, we know more about additives (which make up less than one percent of our diet) than we do about the chemistry of food itself. Food additives, especially those introduced in the past ten years, have survived rigid testing procedures not applied to the great majority of natural products. These tests must prove that the additive is not only safe but performing an important function.

In discussing additives it is important to point out that the same substance can be an additive, a food, or a food ingredient, depending upon how it is used. For example, most sugar is not used as an additive, but much is. If one is eating an after-dinner mint the sugar is the food and the traces of flavor or color that are present are the additives. If one is eating a piece of cake then sugar is an ingredient, it contributes calories and a number of functional values in terms of texture, flavor, lightness, etc. Finally, as a sweetner in a cup of coffee, or fermented in the making of bread, sugar is an additive. In the latter case, it is a yeast food and indirectly a leavening agent.

Whether, in a particular use, sugar or any other substance is primarily a food, an ingredient, or an additive depends on its nature, amount and intent of use. If it is a traditional food or a major source of nutrients, used in relatively large proportion, then it is a food or an ingredient. If it is used in relatively minor amounts, specifically for one or more of the recognized technical effects, then it is an additive. Obviously, the boundaries are not sharp.

In chapter nine of this book we presented a critical review of the report of the McGovern Committee on Dietary Goals because we think it may have an unfavorable effect on U.S. nutritive policies. It is a political report and short on practicability and scientific facts, which unfortunately will not be realized by the vast majority of the many who have received copies.

Contrary to the implications of the report, we believe the U.S. has the best and safest food supply of any country in the world, and the least costly. This is primarily because of the ingenuity of the American food system—agricultural scientists, farmers, the chemical industry, food technologists, food processors, packaging companies, and distributors. Indeed, considering the many facets of industry involved in some aspect of the production and distribution of food, it is by far the largest industry in this country. Despite the constant carping of some of the consumer activists and food faddists, we think the food industry does a remarkably good job in feeding us and much of the world.

The concern about additives—as well as with vitamin regimens and fascinations with quick-weight-loss diets—has to some extent blurred the larger picture of what *is* important in good nutrition. Actually, it is not as complicated as your health-food store owner might lead you to believe. If you are truly interested in eating for good health, forget the latest fads and focus on the three areas which are important and over which you *should* exert control.

1. Variety

As stated earlier, the food one eats is a very personal matter, but the best nutrition is obtained when we eat a variety of foods selected from each of the Basic Four Food Groups and with variety in each of these groups. Menus planned for groups of people may be nutritionally sound in every way, and yet these menus may fail to allow for the fact that one or more of the foods included may not be eaten for cultural or personal reasons. Again, planned but uneaten food serves no nutritional purpose in a diet! Clearly, then, it is necessary to provide a complete easy-to-use guide of wide applicability for the individual to use in planning his daily food intake. The easy-to-use guide is simply variety of food consumption from each of the Basic Four Food Groups. The merits of good nutrition are gaining ever-increasing recognition, but it is the application of this knowledge to daily living that must be achieved.

2. Calories and Salt

While many Americans are worrying about additives, pesticides and "overprocessing" of food, they should be concerned about our number one nutritional problem—overeating. For instance, the National Academy of Sciences suggests that men in the nineteen to twenty-two age group who weigh about 150 pounds need some 3,000 Calories; women in that age group with a weight of about 122-128 pounds may need about 2100 Calories. But calorie needs decline sharply with age.

Obviously, overindulgence in high-calorie "junk food" is not good nutrition (actually a food does not become a "junk food" unless it is overused). Eat moderately, in variety, and this variety can include whatever you consider to be a "junk food." Remember that exercise is an important part of good health, the only way one has of using up calories. One important exercise is pushing away from the table. The best calorie counter we know of is a "bathroom scale" used once a week at the same time of day, say Sunday morning after you have washed but before breakfast. Regardless of your calorie count a consistent weight gain means too many calories for you!

Go easy on the salt shakers. It is an accepted medical fact that excess salt can increase the severity of heart diseases, hypertension and certain kidney diseases. Adding salt to many foods is habit-forming—and it is worth keeping added salt in food to a minimum (all food naturally contains salt).

3. *Fats and Cholesterol*

In everyday terms, control of dietary fat means emphasizing main dishes low in saturated fat such as fish, poultry, and veal instead of a steady diet of beef, using polyunsaturated margarines instead of butter, and eating fewer egg yolks—preferably not more than two or three "visible" eggs (that is, not counting those used in baking and elsewhere) a week. You can "eat to your heart's content," keep your figure and vitality, and reduce your odds on coronary heart disease and some types of cancers by decreasing the total amount of fat in your diet, substituting unsaturated fats including polyunsaturated fats for some of the saturated fat, and decreasing foods rich in cholesterol, particularly egg yolk.

CONCLUSION

There are some fifty known nutrients necessary for the physiologic needs of your body. No single food provides all of these nutrients in adequate amounts, hence, the emphasis on consuming a variety of foods to obtain good nutrition. The psychologic values of foods are provided by taste, smell, color, texture, temperature, and no doubt, countless variations of these factors and others. Again, this emphasizes the importance of variety in the foods we eat.

Nutrition for each individual represents an accumulation of the habits formed throughout one's lifetime. These food preference patterns tend to become increasingly rigid as an individual ages. Dietary patterns vary markedly from individual to individual and from one cultural and geographic environment to another. Food preferences, cultural heritage, and the availability of foods are fundamental in establishing and molding food patterns of individuals. These patterns can be altered, but usually only with considerable effort and patience.

The improvement of the general nutritional status of a population is a long-range goal that can best be achieved through the joint efforts of concerned health and social scientists, educators, agriculturalists, politicians, and consumers. A key to improving the nutrition level in a population is the development of an understanding and appreciation of the psychological and sociological factors determining food consumption patterns. Further progress can be achieved through nutrition education programs intensively directed to students throughout their school years, particularly in the early years. By teaching applied nutrition to children of school age (and even younger), good dietary patterns are encouraged at a time when food habits are being established. Over an extended period of time, such education will begin to influence nutritional habits in all segments of the population.

Appendices

1. *Make Mine Moderate*: A week's menus, averaging 1500 Calories daily, some ideas for reducing that intake down to 1200 Calories and final tips on weight control.
2. *Give Your Heart a Break!*: A week's menus to help you get your cholesterol where it should be and keep it there (by Fredrick J. Stare, M.D. and Patricia S. Remmell, M.S.)
3. *Low-Cholesterol Meals Can Be Elegant*: Seven sample recipes.
4. *Suggested Readings and Sources for Further Nutritional Information.*
5. *Glossary.*
6. *What's Your Nutritional IQ?*
   Quiz Yourself.

Appendix One

Make Mine Moderate:

A week's menus, averaging 1500 Calories daily, some ideas for reducing that intake down to 1200 Calories and final tips on weight control.

"MAKE MINE MODERATE"
A Week's Menus
Moderate in Calories—Moderate in Fat—
Moderate in Cost

Most adults in our country eat too much—too many calories, that is. The ladies are likely to skimp on fruit and dairy products, favoring desserts and breadstuffs. The gentlemen are inclined to emphasize meats and rich foods. Interesting, good-tasting meals can be conservative in calories and in fat, emphasizing the protective foods arranged in what we know may be a "lifesaving" pattern for some.

Now—today—is the time to put into operation yesterday's firm resolutions concerning firm figure control. Remember, you didn't really put on that "spare tire" in one week. You have probably been "working" on it for the past year, or even longer.

Here are a week's menus that can start you on the way to establishing a "conservative" diet pattern. The plans illustrate these points:

1. Good nutrition is common sense.

2. Proper nutritional balance is within the reach of most Americans.

3. Expensive meals are not necessarily more nutritious than low-cost ones. Wise planning—and *variety*, not the size of the grocery bill, is the insurance.

Day One

Moderation is the word to remember in this program: moderate calories, moderate exercise—to which this series of menus adds moderate fat and moderate cost.

Each daily menu provides approximately 1500 Calories if you keep the servings moderate. Fruits and vegetables are figured on the basis of one-half cup as one serving. Meat and entrée dishes are on the basis of three ounces per serving. A glass of milk is eight ounces, one-half cup is four ounces.

Menus for Day One—Approximately 1500 Calories

Breakfast

½ cup orange juice   1 pat margarine
Ready-to-eat cereal with milk   Plain coffee or tea
1 slice whole-wheat toast

10:00 a.m. Coffee Break

Coffee, juice, or nonfat milk

Luncheon Meal

Vegetable soup   2 slices Melba toast
Cottage-cheese salad with to-   Lemon sherbet
   mato and lettuce   Plain tea or coffee

3:00 p.m.

Tea or coffee or carbonated beverage

Dinner Meal

Turkey Cacciatore   Tossed salad with 1 tablespoon
½-cup serving steamed egg   French dressing
   noodles   ½ broiled grapefruit
Braised celery   Plain tea or coffee

Bedtime

1 glass nonfat milk (or a glass of beer)

As for exercise, some form of muscular activity is good for almost everyone. It makes you feel good as well as using up a few calories. By expending 100 or 200 more Calories a day than you did last week, by walking a mile or so, and by some moderation in eating—you are well on your way to success in *Make Mine Moderate*.

Day Two

Variety and imagination: these two concepts can help ensure good nutrition for moderate cost and for moderate calories. Just because we suggest between-meal snacks of nonfat milk is no reason why you have to follow the suggestion every day. A glass of nonfat milk is eighty Calories. So is a small glass of fruit juice, an apple, a soft drink, or a small glass of beer or buttermilk. If you prefer milk with your meals, have your fruit in between.

Menus for Day Two—Approximately 1500 Calories

Breakfast

Stewed prunes
1 soft-boiled egg
1 slice toast

1 teaspoon jelly
Plain coffee or tea

10:00 a.m. Coffee Break

Coffee, juice, or nonfat milk

Luncheon Meal

Peanut-butter-and-lettuce
   sandwich
Jellied vegetable salad

Sliced peaches
Plain tea or coffee

3:00 p.m.

Tea or coffee or carbonated beverage

Dinner Meal

Cranberry-juice cocktail
Baked meat loaf with chili
   sauce
Whipped winter squash

Salad greens with lemon juice
Banana tapioca cream
Plain tea or coffee

Bedtime

1 glass nonfat milk (or a glass of beer)

Don't forget that cocktails have calories too. An ounce of whisky or gin furnishes about 100 Calories, depending on the "proof." And two ounces are twice the calories! If you are serious about your weight, moderation applies to drinks as well as food.

Day Three

You will note that these menus are not difficult to prepare. One need not be graduated from "Le Societé de Cordon Bleu" to cook and serve them attractively. And they have a decided eye to the pocketbook aspect. Yesterday's meatloaf is today's lunch—proper planning—as any well-organized housewife knows.

Liver every couple of weeks is good nutrition and need not be the fancy variety. Lamb liver is a delicate surprise, and good beef liver has a flavor and texture many people really prefer. Chicken and turkey liver supply the same nutrients and provide a nice variety to meals.

Menus for Day Three—Approximately 1500 Calories

Breakfast

½ grapefruit	1 teaspoon jelly
2 strips crisp bacon	Plain coffee or tea
1 slice toast	

10:00 a.m. Coffee Break
Coffee, juice, or nonfat milk

Luncheon Meal

Chicken gumbo soup	Celery sticks
Cold sliced meat-loaf sandwich	Fresh apple
with mustard and lettuce	Plain tea or coffee

3:00 p.m.
Tea or coffee or carbonated beverage

Dinner Meal

Braised liver and onions	Shredded lettuce salad with
Whipped potatoes	lemon
Stewed tomatoes	1 small brownie
	Plain tea or coffee

Bedtime
1 glass nonfat milk (or a glass of beer)

You will notice that we suggest having a "snack" between meals and at bedtime. It need not be milk, but whatever it is, the calories should be figured as part of the total for the day.

Day Four

Now that we are about halfway along in our project—*Make Mine Moderate*—we should remind you that these menus furnish about 1500 Calories a day when moderate servings are used. Most women will lose about one-half to two-thirds of a pound a week. If fewer calories or a little faster weight loss is desired, omit dessert for dinner and/or walk a little farther each day.

Generally speaking, men will lose about one and one-half pounds or so a week. This may be a little too fast for some and not really necessary if your program is one of preventing overweight rather than really slimming. To increase these menus to about 1700 calories a day, make the servings larger and have an extra slice of bread.

Menus for Day Four—Approximately 1500 Calories

Breakfast

½ cup blended juice   1 slice toast
Cooked cereal with raisins and   1 teaspoon jelly
  milk   Plain coffee or tea

10:00 a.m. Coffee Break

Coffee, juice, or nonfat milk

Luncheon Meal

Baked macaroni and cheese   Banana-pineapple cup
Tomato and cucumber salad   Plain tea or coffee
  with oil and vinegar

3:00 p.m.

Tea or coffee or carbonated beverage

Dinner Meal

Broiled filet of haddock with   Chef's salad with French
  lemon butter and parsley   dressing
Mexican corn   Orange ambrosia
Spinach with vinegar   Plain tea or coffee

Bedtime

1 glass nonfat milk (or juice)

We might point out that fish is a very fine food. It supplies high-quality protein, is low in fat—especially the saturated variety—and can be very economical. In fact, it meets all the criteria for moderate menus. Use it often and enjoy its benefits, economic and aesthetic as well as nutritive. Well-prepared fish is a true gourmet delight.

Day Five

One of the moderate considerations in this series of moderate menus is fat. We are fairly convinced that a little common sense as far as intake of fat is concerned is an important health consideration. These menus have fat—butter and margarine, eggs, salad dressing, bacon—the usual high fat foods, but with a difference. The amounts are moderate—only two or three servings a week of each. The salad oils are vegetable, thus adding a good source of unsaturated fatty acids. The meats we suggest are fairly lean.

Naturally, many high-fat foods have to be restricted in menus for calorie-conscious people. Fat foods are high in fat and therefore in calories. Remember, each gram of fat is worth 9 Calories, while a gram of protein or carbohydrate is only 4 Calories—slightly more than a 100 percent difference.

Menus for Day Five—Approximately 1500 Calories

Breakfast

½ cup orange juice   1 teaspoon jelly
Ready-to-eat- cereal with milk   Plain coffee or tea
1 slice toast

10:00 a.m Coffee Break

Coffee, juice, or nonfat milk

Luncheon Meal

Broiled hamburger on a bun   Green pepper and cucumber
   with pickle relish and mus-   sticks
   tard   Fresh pear
     Plain tea or coffee

3:00 p.m.

Tea or coffee or carbonated beverage

Dinner Meal

Broiled frankfurter	Cole slaw
½ cup baked beans	Fruited gelatin dessert
1 slice brown bread	Plain tea or coffee

Bedtime

1 glass nonfat milk (or fruit)

This menu looks pretty traditional. It is. The all-American hamburger and the New Englander's Saturday standby.

You don't have to have franks and baked beans. Franks with mashed potatoes and sauerkraut, or chile con carne are other regional favorites.

Day Six

This menu serves to illustrate the proposition that a typical Sunday family bill of fare can be adapted to the pattern of moderation. The bacon-and-egg breakfast, the Sunday roast with trimmings—even ice cream—all can be enjoyed. The only restriction is on amount. One egg, not two; crisp bacon, not limp; one tablespoon of gravy rather than one-half cup; one-half cup of ice cream rather than one-half pint.

To help keep the menus economical, shop carefully for your meat. The lowest price tag may not mean the best buy. A firm, lean piece of boneless shoulder should give you a delicious Sunday meal and provide leftovers for the next day's stew.

Use fruits in season. Grapefruit and apples are fine in the winter, but in the summer, melon, berries, peaches may be better buys. Canned juices are as nutritious as frozen or fresh. Compare the prices with yields and can contents.

Menus for Day Six—Approximately 1500 Calories

Breakfast

Grapefruit sections	1 slice toast
1 egg, scrambled	1 teaspoon jelly
2 strips crisp bacon	Plain tea or coffee

10:00 a.m. Coffee Break

Coffee, juice, or nonfat milk

Luncheon Meal

Chicken-noodle soup

Fruit-salad plate with banana, pear, peach, ½ cup cottage cheese

1 slice raisin toast with 1 pat butter or margarine

Plain tea or coffee

3:00 p.m.

Tea or coffee or carbonated beverage

Dinner Meal

Vegetable-juice cocktail

Pot roast of beef

Small roasted potato

Browned carrots

Tossed salad with lemon juice

Vanilla ice cream

Plain tea or coffee

Bedtime

1 glass of nonfat milk (or fruit or juice or a glass of beer)

Day Seven

This ends our week of *Make Mine Moderate*. But we hope it doesn't end yours. There is no reason why you can't start all over again, substituting your own favorite dishes and combinations for ours. Just be sure that when you substitute, you do it wisely. Keep the Basic Four in mind and use foods from the same groups with similar caloric value.

Menus for Day Seven—Approximately 1500 Calories

Breakfast

1 small banana, sliced

Cereal (hot or ready-to-eat) with milk

1 slice toast

1 teaspoon jelly

Plain coffee or tea

10:00 a.m. Coffee Break

Coffee, juice, or nonfat milk

Luncheon Meal

Consomme julienne

Grilled cheese sandwich

Lettuce wedge with wine
vinegar dressing

Fruit cup

Plain tea or coffee

3:00 p.m.

Tea or coffee or carbonated beverage

Dinner Meal

Old-fashioned beef stew with
vegetables (made from pot
roast of beef leftovers)

Hard roll

Apple, celery, and escarole
salad with orange-juice
dressing

1 small serving plain sponge
cake

Plain tea or coffee

Bedtime

1 glass of nonfat milk (or fruit or a glass of beer)

Above all, don't confuse moderation with monotony. Repetitious, uninteresting menus can soon put the best of resolutions to rout.

Remember: a before-dinner cocktail must be taken into account. Either eat a little less (no cake) or exercise a little more.

Suggestions For Eating Even Less
(a 1200 Calorie Diet Pattern)

This pattern provides about 1200 Calories for the day. Most women will lose a little more than a pound a week on it. The average man will probably lose about two pounds. It is really too drastic for most men unless your doctor says you must lose weight quickly. Actually, we prefer a reducing diet of about 1500 Calories for the average man.

Breakfast
    Fruit—1 medium serving, fresh or unsweetened canned
    Egg—1, poached or soft boiled
    Toast—1 slice with 1 teaspoon margarine
                         or
    Cereal—½ cup with ¼ cup milk, no sugar
    Coffee or tea—no cream or sugar

11:00 a.m. (or about one hour before lunch)
Nonfat milk or buttermilk—1 glass

Luncheon

Meat (or a substitute for meat)—1 3-ounce portion. Use lean beef, lamb, veal, chicken, fish, plain cottage cheese, cheddar cheese.
Vegetable—1 medium serving; may be raw, as a salad such as lettuce and tomato, or cooked. Use lemon or vinegar for seasoning rather than butter or salad dressings.
Fruit—1 medium serving, fresh or unsweetened canned
Bread—1 slice
Margarine—1 teaspoon or 1 pat
Tea or coffee—no cream or sugar

Mid-afternoon

Iced tea, lemonade, or a Coke

Dinner

Bouillon or consommé or vegetable-juice cocktail—
1 serving
Meat—1 3-ounce portion (see Luncheon)
Potato (or a substitute for potato)—1 small serving of mashed or baked potato, steamed rice, corn, lima beans, or macaroni; or 1 slice bread
Vegetable—1 serving, raw, as a salad, or cooked. *(Note:* One vegetable a day should be a green, leafy one)
Margarine—1 teaspoon, for potato
Fruit—1 medium serving, fresh or unsweetened canned
Tea or coffee—no cream or sugar

Evening or Bedtime

Nonfat milk, buttermilk, soft drink, or glass of beer
Saltines or pretzels—2

Watch your bathroom scales. If you are losing too fast (more than one and one-half pounds a week), add a little to this pattern.

Whole milk in place of nonfat milk	165	Calories
1 cocktail	150	"
1 serving ice cream	150	"
1 piece angel or sponge cake—not iced	150	"
1 ounce cooked meat or 1 egg	80	"
1 serving of cream soup	150	"
10 potato chips	110	"
1 slice bread	60	"
1 pat butter	50	"

If you don't seem to lose, be patient. It may take you a couple of weeks to adjust to the new routine. Don't eat any less. If you have been faithful for about two weeks and nothing happens, think over your activities. Maybe you are not only cutting down on your calories but also on your exercise. Take a short brisk walk twice a day, fifteen minutes or so at a time.

Final Tips on Weight Control

Whatever your own individual caloric needs, and whichever type of diet you choose, it will be useful to keep these tips in mind.

1. Prevention is better than treatment.
2. Early treatment is better than late treatment.
3. Parents should help children develop good food habits by serving (and enjoying) a varied diet and keeping their own weight at the desirable range.
4. Use the bathroom scales—weekly or monthly; and if you have a problem with your weight, keep a written record of it.
5. Eat three or more meals a day, but smaller meals—including a good breakfast; eat in the daytime, not at night.
6. Eat slowly. This allows the blood sugar to rise and satisfy the appetite before it is time for "seconds."
7. Cut down on the total amount of food and on the size of servings. It is not necessary to eliminate any single food.
8. Take your choice between cocktails or dessert.

9. If necessary, use "scientific nibbles,"* not "common nibbles," to help curb your appetite.

10. Take mild to moderate daily exercise.

Please remember that these suggestions are not all documented by firm evidence, but may be helpful to those who have to struggle with the problem of overweight.

---

*Scientific nibbles are part of what you ordinarily would eat with your meal. They are a part of the meal simply eaten in-between meals. Common nibbles are really an "extra".

Appendix Two

Give Your Heart a Break!

A week's menus to help you get your cholesterol where it should be and keep it there. (By Fredrick J. Stare, M.D. and Patricia S. Remmell, M.S.)

There is a growing awareness that the foods we eat, particularly those that provide too much saturated fat and cholesterol, influence our chances of developing coronary heart disease. And because coronary heart disease is the greatest threat to life of adults in this country, we present a special seven-day series on this vital subject—each with a daily menu.

What is the connection between fats in the diet and heart disease? Some kind of fats (the saturated) favor an increase of cholesterol and other fatty substances in the blood. The amount of these substances in the blood, along with other factors, accelerate the development of heart disease. Other kinds of fat, the unsaturated, particularly the polyunsaturated, do the opposite. They tend to decrease the cholesterol in the blood.

Common examples of each type of fat: meat fat, butter, coconut, and palm are largely saturated; safflower, sunflower, soya, corn, and cottonseed are largely polyunsaturated; olive is mostly mono-unsaturated.

The most important way to guard against a rise in blood cholesterol level, or to try and reduce it if it is somewhat elevated, is to eat fewer total calories and pay attention to how much of what foods containing what kinds of fat you eat each day, and to eat fewer egg yolks, as they are the main source of cholesterol in our typical diets.

Such changes are neither drastic nor difficult. They involve putting more emphasis on some foods, less on others. When we speak of "controlling" fat, we mean two things:

- Reducing (not eliminating) the use of foods containing large amounts of fat which is of the saturated type.
- Increasing the use of foods containing large amounts of fat which is of the polyunsaturated type.

We do not mean reducing the total amount of fat in the diet. Later in this series you'll be hearing more about saturates and polyunsaturates as well as cholesterol in foods.

Sound nutrition, good food, and a controlled fat and low-cholesterol diet are all compatible, and that's what we'll discuss and demonstrate.

Here is our first menu.

Day One

Menu for Day One—Approximately 1800 Calories*

Breakfast
Melon wedge or citrus fruit or juice   1 medium serving
Ready-to-eat cereal containing bran   1 serving
Milk for cereal—skimmed or lowfat   ½ cup
Toast   1 slice
Margarine*   1 tsp.
Coffee with milk
Sugar   1 tsp.

Luncheon Meal
Cold sliced turkey—3 slices   3 oz.
Potato salad on lettuce   2/3 cup
Sliced tomato   1 medium
Date bar (made with oil), 2½" x 1½"   1 small serving
Tea or coffee

Dinner Meal

Lamb stew with vegetables, very lean cubes of leg of lamb	3 oz.
Gravy (remove fat from meat juices, thicken, add ½ cup vegetables and seasonings)	½ cup
Steamed potato	1 medium
with margarine*	1 tsp.
Tossed salad	1 serving
with French dressing	1 tbsp.
Baking powder biscuit (with oil)*	1 small
margarine**	1 tsp.
Jellied fruit dessert	½ cup
Tea or coffee	

Snacks

Nonfat milk, or lowfat milk, fruit or juice, soft drink, or beer	1 glass
Cookies (or fruit)	2 (or 1 piece)

*For more calories—somewhat larger servings
*For fewer calories—somewhat smaller servings
**One of the margarines rich in "polyunsaturates"

Day Two

Do you know that a large proportion of the total fat we eat comes from meat?

Meat fat has a lot of saturated fat. Reducing saturates is the key to fat-controlled diets. Special attention must be paid to meat. It is important how often we eat meat and how much at each meal. Plan on having beef, lamb, and pork (or ham) no more than once daily. The cooked weight individual serving portion should not exceed three to four ounces. That is a small serving for a "steak house," but you don't have to eat all that is served at the restaurant, or you can ask for a child's portion. The dog, or you, might enjoy something other than bones in that brown bag you take home.

For the second day of our special series on diets to "manage" cholesterol, we want to mention other ways of helping to keep the amount of saturates in your diet lower. It is most important to pay special attention to meal *selection* and *preparation*. It's not a hard job to do away with the excess fat surrounding a piece of meat. That's easily recognized. But there is a good deal of meat fat hidden within the flesh which cannot be trimmed. It is referred to as "marbling."

First, buy only the cuts of beef, lamb, and pork with a low amount of fat streaking (marbling) throughout the meat. Then—

- Trim easily removable fat from all meat before cooking.
- Trim remaining visible fat before serving or eating.
- Use a rack to allow fat to drain away from meat during roasting or broiling.
- Remove the fat from meat juices, gravies, stews, pot roasts, soups, etc., by one of the two methods: *Chilling* —Let fat solidify in a pan of cold water or in the refrigerator. Remove the hardened fat from meat and/or liquids. *Skimming*—Ladle or draw up with a bulb-type meat baster. Skim fat from surface with a spoon. Blot last few globules of fat with strips of paper toweling.

Still another way to keep saturates down is to use more fish and poultry. They are low in saturated fat and equal to meat in high quality protein.

Chicken broilers or fryers, young turkeys, and cornish hens are excellent choices. Removing the skin and its adhering fat before cooking is a good practice whenever possible. A second best is to trim the skin from poultry at the plate. Poultry lends itself to a delightful variety of recipe preparations. In today's menu, the white sauce for the chicken pie should be made with fat-skimmed stock, canned consomme, or bouillon cubes.

With a few exceptions all kinds of fish—fresh, frozen, smoked, and canned—are good choices. However, breaded precooked frozen fish, seafood, and poultry are not advised since they often have been fried with a saturated-type fat. By adding one of the vegetable oils or some of the polyunsaturated margarines in cooking, we produce a not only favorable, but flavorable main entree item.

Try this recipe for Spicy Flounder Filets. For 2 lbs. flounder or other fish filets, fresh or frozen to serve six: Combine ½ cup oil, ½ cup water, 1/3 cup lemon juice, ¼ cup Worcestershire sauce, ¼ cup grated onion, 2 tbsp. brown sugar, 2 tsp. salt, 1 tsp. powdered mustard, 1 clove garlic, finely chopped, ¼ tsp. pepper, 4 drops liquid hot pepper. Simmer for 5 minutes, stirring occasionally. Cool. Place filets in a single layer in a shallow baking dish. Pour sauce over fish and let stand for ½ hour, turning once. Pour off sauce and reserve for basting while cooking. Broil about 10 minutes, or until surface is browned. Baste with sauce and sprinkle with paprika. Finish cooking in a 350° F. oven for 5 to 10 minutes to cook the fish throughout.

Here is our second menu.

Menu for Day Two—Approximately 1800 Calories*

Breakfast

Sliced banana	½ medium
Ready-to-eat cereal	1 serving
Milk for cereal—skimmed or lowfat	½ cup
Cinnamon toast	1 slice
made with margarine**	1 tsp.
sugar	1 tsp.
cinnamon	
Coffee with milk	
Sugar	1 tsp.

Luncheon Meal

Chicken pie—diced white meat	3 oz.
sauce (chicken stock, milk, flour, vegetables)	½ cup
pastry crust (Stir-'N-Roll pastry) with polyunsaturated oil	1 oz. round
Green pepper cole slaw	1 serving
½ cup shredded cabbage	
1 tbsp. mayonnaise, vinegar, seasonings	
Fresh pear	
Tea or coffee	

Dinner Meal

Broiled spicy flounder filets	4 oz.
Mashed potato	½ cup
with margarine**	1 tsp.
Herb carrots	1 serving
margarine**	1 tsp.
Sliced cucumber salad	1 serving
with oil and vinegar dressing	1 tbsp.
Strawberry-rhubarb cobbler	2/3 cup
(biscuit made with margarine**)	
Tea or coffee	

Snacks

Nonfat milk, or lowfat milk, fruit	1 glass
or juice, soft drink, or beer	
Cookies	2

*For more calories—somewhat larger servings
*For fewer calories—somewhat smaller servings
**One of the margarines rich in "polyunsaturates"

Day Three

Many of our traditional high-protein foods such as beef, pork, and lamb (but not veal, chicken, turkey, or fish) supply a large proportion of saturated fat to our diets. Milk and many of its products, particularly cheese, are also generous in protein and nutritionally superior protein. Milk is an excellent source of calcium, phosphorous, and many of the vitamins. It is really a very nutritious food, but the fat of milk—butter and cream—is a highly saturated fat.

Our markets carry a wide variety of dairy foods, so choose from the assortment wisely when it comes to controlling fat in your diet. Know what dairy foods are high in saturated fat. Some items like cheddar-type and cream cheeses, ice cream, heavy sweet and sour cream have anywhere from five to ten times the proportion of fat, weight for weight, as does whole milk . . . reason enough to eat them sparingly. Use cottage cheese, nonfat and lowfat milks. Products such as yogurt and ice milk are good substitutes for the higher fat items. If you like to drink two or three glasses of milk a day, why not use the lowfat or nonfat (skimmed) variety or buttermilk on occasion? Mixing equal portions of skimmed and whole milk gives a good lowfat milk.

"Filled" milks and creams containing "vegetable fat" have become popular. In these products the butter fat has been removed and replaced by a vegetable fat. Unfortunately, the vegetable fat used is usually coconut oil, and this is just as saturated as butter fat. Many people believe that these products containing vegetable fat are better for their "heart health." They are not. Filled milks, however, may make a valuable contribution to better general nutrition because they usually are less costly, and thus those in the lower income groups can more readily take advantage of the many good nutritive properties of milk. When filled milks are made with one of the polyunsaturated fats, they will make a real contribution to health.

In short, use good judgment when incorporating dairy foods into your menus. No food is taboo . . . it's the amount you eat and how often you eat it that counts.

Today at lunch, a grilled cheese sandwich (made at home with polyunsaturated margarine on the grill) substitutes for meat; ice sherbet rather than a dish of ice cream is the accompanying dessert. For dinner, total saturates are kept low by selecting chicken as the high-protein food. Polyunsaturates are contributed by the margarine, salad dressing, and the cake in which an oil is used instead of shortening.

Balancing fats and having appetizing meals isn't difficult. Why not plan a few lunch and dinner combinations of high-protein entrees for practice at this point?

Here is our third menu.

Menu for Day Three—Approximately 1800 Calories*

Breakfast

Cranberry juice	½ cup
Poached egg	1
Toast	1 slice
Margarine**	1 tsp.
Jelly	½ tbsp.
Coffee with milk	
Sugar	1 tsp.

Luncheon Meal

Tomato soup, diluted with nonfat milk	1 cup
Grilled cheese sandwich	
American cheese	1 slice
bread	2 slices
margarine**	1 tsp.
Citrus section salad	1 serving
with sweet celery-seed dressing	1 tbsp.
Lime sherbet (1/8 quart)	½ cup
Tea or coffee	
Sugar	1 tsp.

Dinner Meal

Broiled breast of chicken	4 oz.
Parsley diced new potatoes	½ cup
with margarine**	1 tsp.
Fresh green beans with basil	½ cup
with margarine**	1 tsp.
Garden salad	1 serving
with French dressing	1 tbsp.
Washington cake	
(2-egg oil cake recipe, using oil)	3 oz. serving
Tea or coffee	

Snacks

Nonfat milk, or lowfat milk, fruit or juice, soft drink, or beer	1 glass
Cookies	2

   *For more calories—somewhat larger servings
   *For fewer calories—somewhat smaller servings
   **One of the margarines rich in "polyunsaturates"

Day Four

Controlling total caloric intake and the type of fat in the diet are the single most important factors in regulating the amount of choles-

terol in the blood, but for Day Four in this special series we are going
to deal primarily with cholesterol-containing foods. Eating less food
rich in cholesterol is also important.

Cholesterol is a fatlike material present in animal foods but not
in vegetable foods. You may not know, but cholesterol is a necessary
substance for the body. Some of the hormones and one of the
vitamins are made from it.

Foods such as eggs, meat, butter, and cheese contain cholesterol.
Fruits, vegetables, nuts, cereals, and grains contain none. Heeding
our previous advice in cutting down on the saturated fats from meat
and dairy foods benefits in another way: it will also help in reducing
the amount of cholesterol eaten.

Why the concern about cholesterol in foods and daily diet? Like
too much saturated fat, too much cholesterol in the diet raises the
blood cholesterol level. It is the level of cholesterol in the blood
which, along with other factors—increase in blood pressure, hereditary
factors, diabetes, cigarette smoking, lack of exercise (or lethargy),
and obesity—accelerates the development of coronary heart disease.

Egg yolks are especially high in cholesterol and a common item of
the diet. We suggest you eat no more than two to three a week. This
number may be used entirely for cooking or baking purposes (cakes,
cookies, puddings, custards, for example) or for a main entree item
(at breakfast: boiled, poached, scrambled egg, or French toast; at
lunch: egg salad sandwich; at supper: omelet, souffle) or for any
combination that one desires. If you're unsure how much egg yolk
you eat in prepared foods, cut the number of "visible" eggs you eat
to only one each week.

There are no limitations on the use of egg whites. Two egg whites
will substitute nicely for one whole egg in most recipes. There is no
such thing as a low-cholesterol egg, at least not yet. But there are
some promising new egg products with less egg yolk and some
egglike products with no egg yolk. Powdered whole dried eggs
diluted with milk solids and soybean protein make excellent scrambled eggs or omelets and yet have much less cholesterol and are
available commercially. Incidentally, these products can be manu-
factured with generous quantities of polyunsaturated fats (ordinary
eggs have very little polyunsaturates).

Organ meats (brains, kidney and liver) rank high in cholesterol.
While you needn't eliminate them from menus, eating them once

every week or two is enough. Certainly a steady diet of one or several of these items is not indicated. We used to think that shellfish (clams, crabs, lobster, scallops, shrimp) were also high in cholesterol, but a few years ago it was found that the analytical method applied to shellfish was inaccurate. When this was corrected, shellfish turned out not to have so much cholesterol. If you can afford them you can have them—in moderation—on a low-cholesterol diet. But don't smother them in melted margarine! And now the menu for today.

Menu for Day Four—Approximately 1800 Calories*

Breakfast	
Fresh grapefruit	½
Ready-to-eat cereal	1 serving
Milk for cereal—skimmed or lowfat	½ cup
Apricot-nut bread (oil recipe)	1 slice
Margarine**	1 tsp.
Coffee with milk	
Sugar	1 tsp.
Luncheon Meal	
Sardine sandwich	3 oz.
rye bread	2 slices
lettuce	
mayonnaise	½ tbsp.
Fresh apple	1 medium
Butterscotch pudding (regular pudding mix and nonfat milk)	½ cup
Tea or coffee	
Dinner Meal	
Bouillon	1 cup
Pot roast of beef—2 thin slices (very lean top of round, trimmed)	3 oz.
Mashed potatoes	1 serving
with margarine**	1 tsp.
Zucchini with onion	1 serving
with margarine**	1 tsp.

Lettuce and tomato salad	1 serving
with French dressing	1 tbsp.
Angel food cake	1 serving
(1/12 of average cake)	
with frozen berries or peaches	1/3 cup
Tea or coffee	

Snacks

Nonfat milk, or lowfat milk,	1 glass
fruit or juice, soft drink,	
or beer	
Cookies	2

    *For more calories—somewhat larger servings
    *For fewer calories—somewhat smaller servings
    **One of the margarines rich in "polyunsaturates"

Day Five

One of the important changes for today's food practices, the fifth of our series, consists of replacing solid fats with the liquid unsaturated vegetable oils. It is true that both solid and liquid vegetable fats are free of cholesterol; however, the vegetable fats naturally hard at room temperature (like coconut oil and cocoa butter) or those sufficiently hardened by hydrogenation (like some shortenings and margarines) are high in saturated fat.

The oils which remain liquid at room temperature—chief among which are the oils of safflower, sunflower, soya, corn, and cottonseed—are our greatest sources of polyunsaturated fat. Use some daily. These oils and the special margarines and shortenings which are low in saturates and high in polyunsaturates are preferred for cooking and baking.

A package label which lists one of the liquid polyunsaturated oils as the first ingredient in margarine is apt to indicate that the margarine is highly polyunsaturated. Not all soft or tub margarines are highly polyunsaturated, though many are. This is one area where our Food and Drug Administration has recently aided the consumer (and physician) with better labeling.

Polyunsaturated vegetable oils may be obtained in the form of mayonnaise and salad dressings, so don't forget to include these in your menus whenever you can. Like the special high polyunsaturated margarines, they can be counted as nearly equal in value where polyunsaturates are concerned.

A food package label listing vegetable oil as an ingredient does not guarantee that it is polyunsaturated oil. On the contrary, most commercial baked goods and prepackaged convenience foods prepared with fat are prepared with a highly saturated vegetable fat—coconut oil. Until baked goods with polyunsaturated oils are available, it's better to open the cookbook and start "from scratch," particularly until the manufacturer identifies on the label the kind of vegetable fat. You'll see that for today's luncheon and dinner desserts we did just that and made our own cake and cookies.

Over the past few days, notice how we've managed to cut down on foods high in saturated fat and to include foods high in polyunsaturated fat. Substitution of polyunsaturates for saturates, *not in addition*, is the key to the fat-controlled diet.

Here is our fifth menu.

Menu for Day Five—Approximately 1800 Calories*

Breakfast

Fresh or frozen orange juice	½ cup
Oatmeal with raisins	½ cup
and brown sugar	2 tsp.
Milk for cereal—skimmed or lowfat	3 oz.
Toast	1 slice
Raspberry jam	½ tbsp.
Coffee with milk	
Sugar	1 tsp.

Luncheon Meal

Baked ham sandwich	2 oz.
—2 thin slices	
bread	2 slices
lettuce	
mayonnaise	½ tbsp.
Pineapple salad—1 large slice	
on lettuce	1 serving
with cottage cheese	2 oz.

Spice cake (2-egg oil cake recipe)   1 serving
   1/12 of a cake, or 3 oz. with 7-
   minute caramel frosting
Tea or coffee

Dinner Meal
Pan-browned filet of haddock   4 oz.
   with margarine**   2 tsp.
   and cocktail sauce   2 tbsp.
Creamed diced potato   1/3 cup
   (sauce made with regular milk
   and 1 tsp. margarine**)
Frozen or fresh broccoli   1 serving
   with lemon
   (with margarine**)   1 tsp.
Escarole and endive salad   1 serving
   with French dressing   1 tbsp.
Old-fashioned sugar cookies   2
   (oil cookbook recipe)
Tea or coffee

Snacks
Nonfat milk, or lowfat milk,   1 glass
   fruit or juice, soft drink,
   or beer
Cookies   2
   *For more calories—somewhat larger servings
   *For fewer calories—somewhat smaller servings
   **One of the margarines rich in "polyunsaturates"

Day Six

Calories can't be avoided in thinking about food selections. A calorie is not a nutrient but a way of measuring the energy supplied by food. If all the calories in the food and drink you consume are not used up in bodily activities, the excess food energy is stored by the body as fat, regardless of the source of the excess calories. Excess calories thus become excess weight in the form of excess body fat and usually in well-recognized places. Maintaining the proper energy balance is still one of the most important health considerations.

You will have noted that all of our menus have been planned at 1800 Calories. Eating and drinking this amount of Calories a day plus a little regular exercise should help most men who are overweight, and most are, to slim down gradually. This number of Calories is not enough for a slender, active person, and it is likely to be too much for the chubby, fairly inactive woman. Calorie adjusting in these menus is not difficult. Follow our examples of either increasing or decreasing the number and size of servings of foods, especially those that are not high in saturated fat. That way you should be able to get your weight where you want it, and then keep it there.

Remember that cocktails add calories—from 100 to 150 per drink. Don't overlook them. Either exercise more or omit the dessert at dinner or the late evening snacks and do the same if you enjoy before-dinner cocktails or an after-dinner highball or glass of beer.

Any diet plan designed for long-term use must meet the recommendations for good nutrition: variety in food selection, balance of nutrients—not only protein, minerals, and vitamins, but fats as well—and balance of calories. The common-sense inclusion of the Basic Four as a guide to good nutrition is all-important in this diet series. Check these menus. Do they supply the following, which are the Basic Four?

- Four or more servings of enriched or whole grain cereals, breads, flour, potato.
- Two or more servings of meat, fish, poultry, dried beans, peas, nuts, or peanut butter.
- Two fruits and two vegetables.
- Two servings of milk, cheese, or other milk products.

Do your menus meet the test? And what size servings? Let the bathroom scales, used once a week, give you that answer.

Here is the menu for today.

Menu for Day Six—Approximately 1800 Calories*

Breakfast
Stewed prunes   ½ cup
Soft-cooked egg   1

Corn muffin (oil recipe)	1
Margarine**	1 tsp.
Jelly	½ tbsp.
Coffee with milk	
Sugar	1 tsp.

Luncheon Meal

Tuna-macaroni salad	
tunafish	½ cup
cooked macaroni	½ cup
mayonnaise	1 tbsp.
celery, pickles, seasonings	
Tomato wedges	3
Raspberry ice milk	½ cup
Melba toast	2 slices
Margarine**	1 tsp.
Tea or coffee	

Dinner Meal

Rare roast top round of beef	4 oz.
2 thin slices	
(well-trimmed of all fat)	
Baked potato	1 medium
with margarine**	1 tsp.
Hearts of lettuce salad	1 serving
with Russian dressing	1 serving
(1 tbsp. mayonnaise)	
Peach crisp (made with	1/3 cup
margarine**)	
Bread	1 slice
Margarine**	1 tsp.
Tea or Coffee	

Snacks

Nonfat milk, or lowfat milk,	1 glass
fruit or juice, soft drink,	
or beer	
Cookies	2

  *For more calories—somewhat larger servings
  *For fewer calories—somewhat smaller servings
  **One of the margarines rich in "polyunsaturates"

Day Seven

This ends our series on menu planning for a controlled-fat diet, one low in saturated fat and cholesterol and high in polyunsaturates. Let us emphasize that we have not referred to a low-fat diet, rather a diet low in saturated fat and high in polyunsaturated fat. It might also be well to emphasize that all fats have the same number of calories.

To continue with our suggestions and your own plans, keep in mind some simple guidelines:

- Plan menus for a week at a time.
- Use lean, well-trimmed beef, lamb, and pork no more often than once daily, and have the serving on the small side.
- Use some form of fish and poultry for other meals, and the servings can be more generous. Other foods such as dry peas, dry beans, and peanut butter can be used to vary menus.
- Choose the lower fat dairy products to replace ones high in fat, such as cottage cheese for cheddar-type cheese; skimmed milk, lowfat milk, or buttermilk for whole milk; milk for heavy cream; and ice milk for ice cream.
- Use liquid oils for salad dressings. Mayonnaise and prepared salad dressings containing no cream or cheese are good substitutes.
- Use one of the oil margarines low in saturated fat and high in polyunsaturates for a table spread and for seasoning vegetables.
- Use one of the polyunsaturated oils or margarines for baking or one of the newer shortenings low in saturates and higher in polyunsaturates.
- Limit consumption of egg yolks to two or three per week to avoid high amounts of food cholesterol.
- Remember that fruits, vegetables, cereals, and bread have very little fat and no cholesterol, and are important to an interesting, well-balanced diet.
- Adjust portion servings so that desired weight is reached and then maintained.
- Alcoholic beverages furnish calories, and don't forget this.

The menu suggestions we have made are not the only way to follow the principles of a controlled-fat diet. Now that you have the principles and examples of menus, use your own ingenuity. If you do, you and yours will have better heart health.

Here is our seventh menu.

Menu for Day Seven—Approximately 1800 Calories*

Breakfast

Orange and grapefruit sections	½ cup
French toast, grilled with oil	1 slice
oil	1 tsp.
syrup	1 tbsp.
Margarine**	½ tsp.
Coffee with milk	
Sugar	1 tsp.

Luncheon Meal

Chicken chow mein	2/3 cup
Steamed rice	½ cup
Sliced pickled beets and onion salad	1 serving
oil and vinegar dressing	1 tbsp.
Butterscotch brownie	1 bar
1/16 of 8" square, made with oil	
Tea or coffee	

Dinner Meal

Consommé julienne	1 cup
Roast loin of pork—3 thin slices (very lean—trim off all fat)	3 oz.
Oven brown potatoes	½ cup
with margarine**	1 tsp.
Frozen mixed vegetables	½ cup
with margarine**	1 tsp.
Chef's salad	1 serving
with Thousand Island dressing	1 tbsp.
Fruit compote	½ cup
Tea or coffee	

Snacks
Nonfat milk, or lowfat milk,   1 glass
   fruit or juice, soft drink,
   or beer
Cookies   2
   *For more calories—somewhat larger servings
   *For fewer calories—somewhat smaller servings
   **One of the margarines rich in "polyunsaturates"

Appendix Three

Low Cholesterol Meals Can Be Elegant:

Seven sample recipes.

1. Tomato Crown Fish

One way to keep your cholesterol low is to serve fish frequently, at least four to six times a week. Try Tomato Crown Fish, a dish that will disprove the old cliche that food which is good for you is usually dull.

To prepare this dish, freshen 1½ pounds of fish filet (we suggest sliced haddock) for several minutes in a mixture of 1½ cups of water and 2 tablespoons of lemon juice. Then place the fish filet in a greased baking dish and season lightly. Slice 2 large fresh or canned whole tomatoes and place on the fish. Then sprinkle with ½ green pepper, minced, and 2 tablespoons minced onion. Mix ½ cup of bread crumbs, 1 tablespoon of polyunsaturated oil, and ½ teaspoon of basil. Sprinkle the crumb mixture evenly over the vegetables. Bake 10-15 minutes in a 350° oven.

Serve with slightly undercooked, frozen peas mixed with cooked rice. Sprinkle lightly with monosodium glutamate and pepper.

2. Country Baked Chicken

Chicken is a wise choice because it's low in fat, and the fat in chicken has a higher proportion of the polyunsaturated fats than many meats. Since it's low in fat, it's also low in calories.

To make four servings of Country Baked Chicken, quarter one chicken. Wash and dry the chicken pieces carefully. Dip the chicken first in a mixture of ½ cup of polyunsaturated vegetable oil or melted polyunsaturated margarine, ½ teaspoon grated lemon peel, and 3 tablespoons of lemon juice. Then roll the chicken in seasoned cracker, bread, or cereal crumb mixture until the chicken is well-coated. Place the chicken skin side up in a baking pan in a moderate oven (350°F.) for forty-five minutes or until the chicken is tender and well-browned.

If you wish, rub small peeled potatoes with seasoned polyunsaturated vegetable oil and roast with the chicken. To complete the meal, serve your favorite green vegetable and as an accent a colorful molded fruit salad.

3. Barbequed Chicken

There is nothing simpler or more fun than cooking on the backyard barbeque. Best of all, no pots or pans are required. Here is the way our barbequed chicken is prepared. For four persons take one nice, plump, quartered chicken. Season lightly with paprika and cayenne pepper. The chicken is now ready to cook. For the barbeque sauce blend together 4 tablespoons of vegetable oil, 4 tablespoons of honey and 2 tablespoons of lemon juice. Remove 2 tablespoons of this sauce, add to it 1 tablespoon of toasted sesame seeds, and set aside for later use. Baste the chicken with the barbeque sauce while it cooks. Just a few minutes before serving, spoon ½ tablespoon of the sesame sauce over each chicken quarter.

Our vegetable combination is sometimes called a Hobo Special. For each person, wrap in a square of tinfoil a nice clean carrot, a scrubbed potato and a peeled onion and season lightly. Add 1 tablespoon of one of the soft margarines (which are low in saturated fat and relatively high in the polyunsaturates) and a tablespoon of chicken broth. Seal the foil tightly around the vegetables and place in the coals of the fire while the chicken cooks. If you wish, serve a green salad tossed with your favorite oil and vinegar dressing and French garlic bread. Watermelon with lots of napkins adds the right touch for dessert.

A word of caution—weight watchers in the family should choose small or moderate sized servings and have either bread or potato, not both. Watermelon, a delicious low-calorie dessert, can be enjoyed by all.

4. *Veal Supreme*

The recipe, Veal Supreme, is a "put together in the morning and cook in the evening" favorite. If you like—and it tastes even better this way—cook it in the morning and just heat it for dinner. Sprinkle four veal steaks lightly with salt and pepper and brown in a poly-unsaturated oil (corn, soya, cottonseed, or safflower). Place the veal in a casserole. Now saute 12 mushrooms or one small can of mushrooms and 3 onions chopped very fine for several minutes, add a can of mushroom soup diluted with ½ cup broth, and the juice of ½ lemon. Blend well and pour the sauce over the veal. Cook in a tightly covered casserole in a moderate oven (350°F.) for about an hour or until the steaks are tender. About ten minutes before serving add 8 cooked baby onions and, for color, several cooked sliced carrots. Serve very hot.

With the veal serve parsleyed rice and a nice crisp salad with your favorite oil dressing. For dessert, have any of the delicious fresh fruits in season—perhaps a honeydew melon served with several red ripe strawberries, a few plump purple grapes, and a slice of lemon or lime.

This menu is good for heart health because the proportion of saturated to unsaturated fat is pointed in the right direction. Veal is lower in fat and calories than many other meats, therefore, the amount of saturated fat is reduced. Polyunsaturated oil is used in the veal recipe and to dress the salad to help provide a healthful balance of fats.

Fruits are just the right dessert; their low calorie content makes them a wise choice for the millions of Americans who must watch their weight. Besides, they are nutritious and delicious. The colorful combination of fruits suggested adds eye appeal to this meal to help make eating a real pleasure.

5. *Baked Fish Provencale*

To serve four, freshen four fish filets by immersing them in a mixture of equal parts lemon juice and water for a few minutes. Place the filets in an oiled baking dish and season lightly with mono-sodium glutamate, pepper, and powdered garlic. Sprinkle fish with 2 tablespoons of lemon juice and ¼ teaspoon of dill weed. Barely cover fish with skimmed milk (make your own from powdered milk if you like), and top each filet with a slice of onion and a slice of lemon. Sprinkle with chopped parsley. Cover baking dish with a lid or aluminum foil and bake in a moderate (325°F) oven about thirty minutes. If you like, serve with baby carrots seasoned with brown sugar and powdered ginger to taste.

A delightful salad to try with this fish is Romaine lettuce with a simple oil and vinegar dressing. Whipped orange jello topped with mandarin orange sections would provide the proper gourmet finish.

6. *Sweet and Sour Pork*

Sweet and Sour Pork is keyed to heart health with a gourmet flair. Since many pork cuts are high in fat and hence in calories, we reserve it for special occasions and to allow variety. When you use pork, select cuts which have less fat, such as pork loin, and trim off the excess fat before using.

To prepare the Sweet and Sour Pork, trim all visible fat from 1½ pounds of lean pork roast and cut it in thin strips. Saute the meat in 2 tablespoons of polyunsaturated vegetable oil until golden brown, then set aside. Combine the juice drained from a can of pineapple chunks with ½ cup water, 1/3 cup vinegar, ¼ cup brown sugar, 2 tablespoons cornstarch, and salt and soy sauce to taste. Shake in a covered glass jar until well-mixed and then cook over medium heat until clear and slightly thickened. Add the meat and simmer over low heat for about one hour. About five minutes before serving add 3/4 cup of thinly sliced green pepper, ½ cup of onion, sliced thin, and the pineapple chunks. Spoon over hot steamed cooked rice. To make this a real Chinese meal, serve with hot tea and as a special treat have fortune cookies for dessert.

7. *Chicken a l'Orange*

It looks as good as it tastes. First, take one nice cut-up plump fryer and drop these chicken pieces into a mixture of ½ cup of flour, ½ teaspoon of salt, 2 teaspoons of grated orange peel, 1 teaspoon of paprika, and ½ teaspoon of pepper. Toss them well until they are all covered with the flour mixture. Put 2 tablespoons of the seasoned flour mixture aside for the gravy.

Brown the chicken over low heat in 1 tablespoon of margarine until it's golden on all sides. Add ½ cup of water and simmer this gently for about thirty minutes. Turn occasionally and add a little bit more water if necessary. Remove the chicken to a warm platter and pour off the drippings, reserving only 2 tablespoons of the drippings and return these to the skillet with the 2 tablespoons of your flour mixture. Blend it well and then combine 2 cups of orange juice, 2 tablespoons of brown sugar, ¼ teaspoon of ground ginger, 1/8 teaspoon cinnamon and cook this until the mixture boils. Serve this gravy over the chicken. Ground pecan nuts on top of the chicken is an especially elegant touch. Serve the chicken with a nice dry rice.

For our vegetable—saute some cooked green beans in margarine along with a pinch of pepper, some chopped parsley, and a little garlic powder.

Our dessert is Bananas Flambe. Sprinkle peeled bananas with 1 tablespoon of sugar. Place the bananas on a lightly oiled pie plate. Bake them for twenty minutes at 400 degrees, or until they are slightly brown. Flame your bananas by placing a cube of sugar that has been immersed in lemon extract on top of the bananas and light with a match at the table. This is the gay touch that your family and your guests will appreciate, and remember your family's heart health is your concern.

And keep the portions of everything reasonable!

Appendix Four

Suggested Readings and Sources for
Further Nutritional Information

GENERAL REFERENCES ON FOOD

Deutsch, R. *The Family Guide to Better Food and Better Health.* Des Moines, Iowa: Meredith Corp., 1971.

Deutsch, R. *Realities of Nutrition*, Bull Publishing Co., 1976.

Eat to Live, 1976 edition. Wheat-Flour Institute (1776 "F" Street, Washington, D.C. 20006).

Food Is More Than Just Something to Eat. Food and Drug Administration (5600 Fishers Lane, Rockville, MD 20852).

Food of Our Fathers. Institute of Food Technologists, Chicago.

Latham, M.C. et al. *Scope Manual on Nutrition*, 3rd edition. Kalamazoo, Michigan: The Upjohn Company, 1975.

Lowenberg, M., E. N. Todhunter, E. D. Wilson, J. R. Savage and J. L. Lubawski. *Food and Man.* 1974.

National Academy of Sciences. *Recommended Dietary Allowances*, 8th edition. Washington, D.C. 1974.

"Nutrition in the Causation of Cancer" (Part 2 of two parts), *Cancer Research* 35: November, 1975.

Robinson, C. H. *Basic Nutrition and Diet Therapy.* MacMillan, 1975.

Stare, F. J. and McWilliams, M. *Living Nutrition*, 2nd edition. New York: John Wiley and Sons, Inc. 1977.

Stare, F. J. and E. M. Whelan. "The Best Diet for You and Your Health" *Health Values* 1:27, 1977.

Stare F. J. and McWilliams, M. *Nutrition For Good Health*, Plycon Press, 1974.

White, P. L., editor, *Let's Talk About Food*, 2nd edition. The American Medical Association, 1974.

FOOD FADDISM

Barrett, S. and G. Knight. *The Health Robbers*. Philadelphia: George F. Stickley Co., 1976.

Deutsch, R. *The New Nuts Among the Berries*. Bull Publishing, 1977.

"Food Facts Talk Back". The American Dietetic Association, 1975.

Rynearson, E. H. "Americans Love Hogwash", *Nutrition Reviews* (supplement), July 1974.

Trager, J. *The Bellybook*. New York: Grossman, 1972.

WEIGHT CONTROL

"The Healthy Way to Weigh Less". The American Medical Association, 1973.

Ferguson, J., *Habits Not Diets*, Bull Publishing Co., 1976.

Jordan, H. A., Levitz, L. S. and Kimbrell, G. M. *Eating Is Okay: A Radical Approach to Successful Weight Loss*. Rawson Assoc. 1976.

Konishi, F. *Exercise Equivalents of Foods*. Southern Illinois University Press, 1974.

Redbook's Wise Woman's Diet and Exercise Book. McCall Publishing Co., 1970.

Schanche, D. "Diet Books That Poison Your Mind and Harm Your Body." *Today's Health*, April 1974.

Schoenberg, H. *Cookbook for Calorie Watchers*. Good Housekeeping Books, 1972.

Siegel, M. J. and D. Van Keuren. *Think Thin*. New York: Paul S. Eriksson Inc., 1971.

Stare, F. J. and E. M. Whelan. "Rating the Diets." *Harper's Bazaar*, July 1977.

Stuart, R. and B. Davis. *Slim Chance in a Fat World*. Champaign, Illinois: Research Press, 1972.

FOOD ADDITIVES/PESTICIDES/"CHEMICALS"

Benarde, M. A. *The Chemicals We Eat*. New York: American Heritage Press, 1971.

Food & Nutrition Board. *Toxicants Occurring Naturally in Foods*. Washington D. C.: National Academy of Sciences, 1973.

Jukes, T. H. "Nutrition and the Food Supply: Controversies and Prospects." *American Biology Teacher* 38 (1976): 162.

Whelan, E. M. and F. J. Stare. *Panic in the Pantry: Food Facts, Fads and Fallacies*. New York: Atheneum, 1977.

White, P. L. and D. Fletcher, eds. *Nutrients in Processed Foods: Vitamins & Minerals*. Acton, Mass.: Publishing Sciences Group, Inc., 1974.

INFANT AND CHILD CARE

Fomon, S. J. *Infant Nutrition*. 2nd edition. Philadelphia: W. B. Saunders Co., 1975.

DIABETES

Dolger, H. and B. Seeman. *How to Live with Diabetes*. 3rd edition. New York: W. W. Norton and Co., 1972.

Duncan, T. and others. *The Good Life with Diabetes*. Philadelphia, Pa.: The Garfield G. Duncan Research Foundation, Inc., 1973.

Fischer, A. and D. Horstmann. *A Handbook for Diabetic Children*. New York: Intercontinental Medical Book Corp., 1972.

Gormican, A. *Controlling Diabetics with Diet*. Springfield, Illinois: Charles C. Thomas, 1971.

HEART DISEASE AND DIET

Cutler, C. *Haute Cuisine for Your Heart's Delight*. New York: Clarkson N. Potter, 1973.

Eshleman, R. and M. Winston. *The American Heart Association Cookbook*. New York: David McKay Co., Inc., 1973.

Keys, A. and M. Keys. *How to Eat Well and Stay Well the Mediterranean Way*. Garden City, New York: Doubleday, 1975.

Margolese, R. G. *A Doctor's Eat-Hearty Guide for Good Health and Long Life*. Englewood Cliffs, New Jersey: Prentice Hall, 1974.

LOW SODIUM DIET

Bagg, E. W. *Cooking Without a Grain of Salt*. New York: Doubleday, 1964.

Payne, A. S. and D. Callahan. *The Fat and Sodium Control Cookbook*. Revised. Boston: Little, Brown and Co., 1965.

FLUORIDATION

"Fluoridation Facts." Chicago: American Dental Association, 1974.
Maier, F. *Fluoridation*. Cleveland, Ohio: CRC Press, 1972.

SOURCES OF NUTRITION-EDUCATIONAL MATERIALS

1. *Colleges and Universities* – Departments of Home Economics, Biochemistry and Nutrition

2. *Food Industries* – Departments of Home Economics and Public Relations

3. *Nutrition Foundation* – Office of Education and Public Affairs, 888 Seventeenth Street, N.W., Washington, D.C.

4. *Government Agencies*:

   Food and Drug Administration
   Department of Health, Education and Welfare
   5600 Fishers Lane, Rockville, Maryland 20852

   National Academy of Sciences, National Research Council
   Food and Nutrition Board
   2101 Constitution Avenue, Washington, D. C.

   National Institutes of Health
   U. S. Public Health Service, Bethesda, Maryland

   Superintendent of Documents
   U. S. Government Printing Office, Washington, D. C. 20402

   Also, state and local health departments

5. *National Professional Organizations*:

   American Medical Association, Dept. of Food and Nutrition
   535 North Dearborn Street, Chicago, Illinois 60610

American Dietetic Association
430 North Michigan Avenue, Chicago, Illinois 60611

American Dental Association
211 East Chicago Avenue, Chicago, Illinois 60611

American Geriatrics Society
10 Columbus Circle, New York, N. Y. 10010

Society for Nutrition Education
2140 Shattuck Avenue, Suite 1110
Berkeley, California 94704

Nutrition Today
101 Ridgely
Annapolis, Maryland 21404

Institute of Food Technologists
221 North La Salle Street, Chicago, Illinois 60601

6. *Trade Associations:*

Cereal Institute
1111 Plaza Dr., Schaumburg, Illinois 60195

Manufacturing Chemists Association
1825 Connecticut Avenue, N.W., Washington, D.C. 20009

National Dairy Council
6300 North River Rd., Rosemont, Illinois 60018

7. *Voluntary Health Organizations*: (National and Local Chapters)

American Diabetes Association
One West 48th Street, New York, N. Y. 10020

American Heart Association
7320 Greenville Ave., Dallas, Texas 75321

The Arthritis Foundation
221 Park Ave, South, New York, N. Y. 10003

Appendix Five

Glossary

Adipose: A medical term meaning fatty. Usually used in reference to the animal tissue that stores fat—as, adipose tissue.

Amino Acids: The basic chemical compounds that when properly combined make up proteins—the building blocks of proteins. They are organic compounds containing nitrogen as well as carbon, hydrogen, and oxygen. There are some twenty-two amino acids, eight of which are called "essential" because the body cells cannot make them and hence it is essential that they be received from the foods of the diet. The other amino acids are also obtained from foods, but the body can also make them, principally in the liver, from other dietary ingredients.

Anemia: A blood disorder in which there is either an insufficient number of red blood cells or a reduced amount of hemoglobin, the oxygen-carrying pigment of the red blood cells, or both.

Arteriosclerosis: A thickening and occasionally a hardening, due to calcification, of the walls of arteries and capillaries resulting in a loss of elasticity of the vessel wall and a narrowing of the size of the vessel.

Ascorbic Acid: Another name for vitamin C, the vitamin historically associated with the disease called scurvy. Ascorbic acid is particularly necessary for healthy gums, as well as many other body tissues, because of its role in the formation of connective tissue. Fresh fruits (especially citrus) and vegetables are the principal sources of this vitamin.

Atherosclerosis: A type of arteriosclerosis characterized by fatty deposits containing cholesterol in the inner lining of arteries. It is

303

the type of arteriosclerosis usually present when one has coronary heart disease, a stroke, or an aneurysm.

Balanced Diet: A diet made up of a variety of foods from the different food groups (Basic Four) so that all the many nutrients are obtained in proper or balanced amounts.

Basic Four: A term used to describe a classification of foods into four groups that supply certain categories of nutrients:

> 1. The meat group
> 2. The milk group
> 3. The vegetable-and-fruit group
> 4. The bread-and-cereal group

By eating certain quantities of foods from each group one is likely to receive a "balanced diet"—that is, a diet providing all nutrients in proper amounts.

Bioflavonoids: Compounds found in citrus fruits and often associated with ascorbic acid. The biological importance of these substances, if any, is not known.

Bran: The coarse outer coat of grains. In the diet it provides bulk, and this is important to prevent constipation.

Calcium: A mineral nutrient, essential for bone and teeth formation, and a variety of metabolic processes such as the clotting of blood, beating of the heart, and other types of muscular contraction, and the conduction of impulses along nerve fibers.

Calorie: The unit by which the energy value of food is measured. The calorie, or energy value of foods, is defined as the amount of heat energy required to raise 1000 grams (approximately one quart) of water one degree Centigrade. In practice, the calorie value is determined by calculation using the composition of the food in terms of fat, protein, and carbohydrate. Each gram of fat produces nine Calories, and each gram of protein and carbohydrate, four Calories.

Carbohydrate: A group of organic chemical substances containing carbon, hydrogen, and oxygen that are found in foods and utilized by the body for energy. Starch and sugars are the common carbohydrates. Cereals and root vegetables are the common food sources of starches.

Caries: Tooth decay.

Carotene: A yellow compound of carbon and hydrogen found in yellow and green plants and converted by the body into vitamin A. In green plants the yellow color is masked by a larger concentration of the green pigment known as chlorophyll.

Cell: The structural and functional microscopic unit of plant and animal organisms.

Cellulose: A complex carbohydrate found in the fibrous parts of plants. It is poorly digested by humans and hence provides no calories. Cows, sheep, goats, and horses can digest cellulose and get energy from it.

Cesium 137: The radioactive form of the mineral element cesium.

Chemical: A chemical is any substance made up of elements. For example, two atoms of hydrogen and one of oxygen make a molecule of water (H_2O)—a chemical. One atom of sodium and one of chlorine make a molecule of table salt (NaCl)—a chemical. A number of atoms of hydrogen, oxygen, and carbon when combined in the proper way make a molecule of cholesterol, and thousands of other chemicals.

Cholesterol: The commonest member of a group of compounds called "sterols." These are composed of carbon, hydrogen, and oxygen. Cholesterol is present in all animal tissues but not in plant tissues, though the latter contain similar sterols. Cholesterol is present in many foods, but only foods of animal origin. Egg yolk, sweetbreads, liver, brains, and shellfish are especially rich sources. It is also made by the body. It is an essential raw material for the manufacture by the body of sex and adrenal hormones, of vitamin D, and is a constituent of the abnormal deposits in the inner layer of arteries giving rise to atherosclerosis.

Colitis: Inflammation of the colon, which is the wider part of the intestine making up the latter half of this organ.

Coronary: Referring to the arteries within the heart and which supply the heart muscle tissue with nourishment and oxygen.

Deficiency Disease: A disease resulting form the inadequate intake (a deficiency) of an essential nutrient. Thus scurvy is due to a deficiency of ascorbic acid, pellagra to a deficiency of niacin, and kwashiorkor to a deficiency of protein.

Dentin: The portion of the tooth beneath the enamel and surrounding the tooth pulp.

Desirable Weight: That weight at which most people will live longest. Insurance actuarial data indicate that average weight at age twenty-five years for each sex and for any given height is best for longevity, and the Metropolitan Life Insurance Company termed this "desirable weight." Prior to about 1945 this weight was called "ideal weight."

Digestion: The breaking down of foods into simple components in the digestive tract and their absorption into the blood. Proteins are digested to peptides and amino acids, fats to fatty acids and glycerol, and carbohydrates to dextrins and sugars.

Edema: An accumulation of abnormal amounts of fluid in the inter-tissue spaces of the body, between cells, which results in a swelling.

Edible: A term applied to that portion of food that is fit (or ready) to eat.

Element: Any one of the atoms of which all matter is composed.

Emulsification: The process of breaking large fat particles into smaller ones that will remain suspended as small particles in another liquid— as, for example, the small particles of fat suspended in homogenized milk.

Endocrine: A term applied to organs that secrete directly into the blood a substance or substances called hormones, which regulate various phases of metabolism.

Endogenous: A term used to refer to substances originating from within or inside the cells or tissues as contrasted with substances reaching tissues from outside the body. Thus endogenous cholesterol refers to the cholesterol manufactured by the body out of other compounds, and exogenous cholesterol refers to cholesterol obtained from foods.

Energy: In nutrition the caloric equivalent of the heat and work necessary to maintain the temperature of the body and permit muscular contraction and thus perform work.

Enrich: To add one or more nutrients to a food to bring its content of those nutrients up to the approximate level in the food before processing.

Enzyme: A substance, protein in nature, formed in living cells, which brings about and greatly accelerates chemical changes but does not enter into the change. Many enzymes consist of specific vitamins combined with specific proteins.

Essential: A term used to refer to specific nutrients required for some body reactions essential to life and which must be supplied from foods because the body cannot make these nutrients from other dietary substances. Thus, lysine is an "essential" amino acid essential for growth, and must be received in adequate amounts from the diet; however, glycine, another amino acid, is not essential in the diet, as the body can make it from other components of the diet. Copper and iron are mineral nutrients essential for the formation of hemoglobin, the red coloring matter of the blood that is needed to carry oxygen to the cells of the body, obviously an essential function. Fluoride is a mineral nutrient essential for the formation of dental enamel that has a chemical and physical structure that provides maximum resistance to decay.

Exogenous: A term used to refer to substances originating outside the cells or tissues of the body. For example: exogenous cholesterol refers to dietary sources of cholesterol, not that made within the body, which is called endogenous (q.v.).

Fat: A chemical compound composed of three fatty acids combined with a molecule of glycerol. Fats are either animal or vegetable in origin and may be solid or liquid. They also may be man-made—that is, synthesized in the laboratory.

Fat Soluble: Refers to substances that do not dissolve in water but do in fats, oils, or in fat solvents. For example, vitamins A and D are fat soluble. In nature they are found dissolved in butterfat, as contrasted with vitamin C, which is water soluble and found dissolved in the watery juice of citrus fruit.

Fatty Acids: Organic acids that combine with glycerol to form fat. They are usually classified as "saturated" or "unsaturated." Fatty acids are chains of carbon atoms to which are attached two hydrogen atoms for each carbon atom, and at the end of the chain are two oxygen atoms, one combined with carbon and the other with carbon and hydrogen. If all the hydrogens that can be attached to the carbon atoms are present in the chain, the acid is called saturated. If two adjacent carbons are each lacking a hydrogen, a "double bond" results and the acid is considered unsaturated—that is, hydrogen can be added at the site of the double bond. If there is one double bond in the chain the fatty acid is called monounsaturated. Olive oil is an example of an oil containing a good deal of monounsaturated fatty acid, the specific acid being oleic acid. If there are two or more double bonds the substance is called polyunsaturated. The most common polyunsaturated fatty acid (pufa) is called linoleic acid. It is found in corn, cottonseed, safflower, soy oil, where it makes up about half or more of the total fatty acids. Linoleic acid is an "essential" fatty acid since it must be furnished by the food we eat. Linolenic and arachidonic are two other polyunsaturated fatty acids that are "essential."

Fluoridation: The adjustment of the mineral nutrient fluoride in a water supply, usually so that the concentration of fluoride will be one part of fluoride per million parts of water. Fluoridation is a public-health procedure that will reduce the amount of dental decay in children, and future adults, by 60 to 70 percent.

Folic Acid: A vitamin of the B-complex group, and important in metabolism of the red blood cells and in certain enzyme reactions.

Food Additives: Chemical compounds added to foods to improve flavor, appearance, preservation, or nutritive qualities and thus provide better nutrition and economy through longer keeping qualities of the food.

Food Faddist: One who attaches unusual health-promoting properties to a specific food or diet, usually for a specific disease or group of diseases, and in the absence of any generally accepted scientific evidence.

Food Quack: One who pretends to know something about foods and nutrition, generally in relation to human health, but who has had little or no training in these subjects and who is not recognized or respected by those who have studied and contributed to this area of science.

Fortify: To add one or more nutrients to a food so that it contains more of the nutrient than the food provides as it occurs in nature. For example, milk is often fortified with vitamin D, and margarines with vitamin A.

Galactose: A simple sugar derived from milk sugar or lactose, it constitutes half of the molecule of lactose.

Gliadin: One of the proteins found in wheat.

Glucose: A simple sugar that makes up half of the molecule of sucrose, which is ordinary table sugar. It is also the type of sugar present in the blood and which is utilized (metabolized) by the body to yield energy.

Gluten: A protein found in many cereal grains.

Gram: A unit of weight in the metric system. One gram is approximately 1/28 of an ounce.

Iodine: A mineral nutrient essential for the proper functioning of the thyroid gland as it is a part of the molecule of the hormone thyroxin which is made by this endocrine gland.

Iron: A mineral nutrient, necessary for the formation of hemoglobin, the substance in red blood cells necessary for carrying oxygen to the cells of the body.

Kwashiorkor: The name of a disease occurring in children generally between one and five years of age in many of the underdeveloped areas of the world. It is due to lack of adequate quantities of good quality protein, is frequently a fatal disease, and is one of the leading causes of death in this age group in underdeveloped countries.

Linoleic Acid: *See* fatty acids.

Linolenic Acid: *See* fatty acids.

Lipid: Fat or fatlike substances.

Metabolism: A term used to describe all chemical changes that occur in living matter.

Milligram: A measure of weight in the metric system, 1/1000 of a gram.

Minerals: Naturally occurring inorganic elements, some of which are essential to life in animals and plants. The minerals commonly given consideration in human nutrition are sodium, potassium, calcium, phosphorus, iron, iodine, copper, magnesium, cobalt, chlorine, manganese, fluorine, sulfur, selenium, zinc, and molybodenum.

Niacin: A member of the B-complex vitamins. Historically, it is associated with the prevention of pellagra.

Nutrient: A chemical compound needed for specific functions in the nourishment of the body. Protein, amino acids, fat, sugar, starch, minerals, vitamins, water are all nutrients. There are some fifty known nutrients.

Obesity: Excessive body weight due to the presence of a surplus of body fat, sometimes defined as 20 percent or more above "desirable" weight.

Oils: Any fat that remains liquid at room temperature. Most of the common edible oils are of vegetable origin and contain a fair supply of monounsaturated or polyunsaturated fatty acids.

Overweight: Sometimes defined as 10 to 20 percent over "desirable" weight, as contrasted with obese, which is 20 percent or more above "desirable" weight.

Phenylketonuria: A hereditary disease in which there is a lack of the specific enzyme needed to use (metabolize) the amino acid phenylalanine. This disease results in an increased amount of phenylpyruvic acid in the blood and urine and may damage parts of the brain, causing mental retardation. The disease is usually diagnosed in infancy or early childhood.

Radionuclide: A radioactive atom in which the nucleus of the atom has become radioactive naturally or by the use of atomic energy.

Riboflavin: A water-soluble vitamin of the B-complex that is important in many enzyme reactions, particularly those involving the transfer of energy from food to the cells.

Roughage: The indigestible material found in food. In vegetables, it is called cellulose, bran, or fiber; in animals, it is connective tissue.

Saccharin: A white crystalline compound of high degree of sweetness used as a substitute for sugar. It has no caloric value.

Serum: The colorless fluid portion of the blood that separates when the blood cells are removed by clotting or centrifugation.

Sodium: A mineral nutrient involved in many of the fluid systems of the body. The most common food source is table salt, which makes up about half the molecule by weight.

Sterol: Fatlike or fat-soluble compounds with a somewhat complex structure. Cholesterol and vitamin D are common examples of the sterols.

Strontium-90: The radioactive form of the element strontium.

Synthetic: Refers to the process of making or "building up" a compound by the union of simpler compounds or their elements. Common usage assigns this term to compounds made in the laboratory, or in industry, as opposed to compounds made by the body.

Thiamine: One of the B-complex vitamins, also known as vitamin B_1. Historically, it is associated with the prevention of the disease known as beriberi, which is common among those who eat large amounts of polished rice.

Tooth Enamel: The hard outer covering of the tooth made of inorganic material, mostly complex compounds of calcium and phosphates, and which is made more resistant to decay when fluoride is combined with the calcium and the phosphates.

Vascular: Pertaining to, or full of, blood vessels.

Vitamin: One of a group of substances that in relatively small amounts are essential for life and growth. They are commonly divided into two groups on the basis of their solubility: the fat-soluble vitamins (A, D, E, and K); and the water-soluble vitamins (ascorbic acid or vitamin C and the B-complex vitamins).

Vitamin A: A member of the fat-soluble vitamins. It is necessary for growth, vision, and healthy skin. Carotene (q.v.), a yellow pigment in fruit and vegetables, is a precursor of vitamin A, in that in the body it is converted into vitamin A.

Vitamin B Complex: *See* individual B-vitamins—thiamine, riboflavin, niacin, and folic acid.

Vitamin C: *See* ascorbic acid.

Vitamin D: A fat-soluble vitamin—the "sunshine vitamin," important for building strong bones and teeth in that it favors the absorption of calcium. We usually get all we need by the action of sunlight in changing certain sterols in the skin into vitamin D. This is then transported by the blood to the liver, where it is stored for future use.

Vitamin K: A fat-soluble vitamin needed for the clotting of blood. There are no good food sources of vitamin K. Most of it is obtained by absorbing it from bacteria that normally live and multiply in your large intestine.

Appendix Six

What's Your Nutritional IQ? Quiz Yourself

(Questions with the Answers on the Following Pages)

1. Is it true that Americans
   a. are well-nourished?
   b. are overnourished?
   c. are ill-fed?
   d. were well-nourished but are getting worse all the time?

2. What effect does pasteurization of fresh milk have on its nutritive value?
   a. Increases it.
   b. Decreases it.
   c. Does not change it at all.

3. How does canned (evaporated) milk compare to the whole fresh product as a milk source for youngsters?
   a. As good as fresh milk.
   b. Better than fresh milk.
   c. Inferior to fresh milk.

4. How well informed are you about some of the following nutritional requirements of young babies?
   A. The first week or two after birth, a normal baby needs per day about
   1. 25 Calories per pound.
   2. 35 Calories per pound.
   3. 45 Calories per pound.
   B. In this country a common nutritional deficiency is that of infantile anemia, which appears in the latter half of the first year. In order to prevent this, a food source of iron should be given by
   1. Six weeks of age.
   2. Three months of age.
   3. Six months of age.
   C. Protein is needed for the proper growth and development of a baby. The needs are high at this period because the young infant's growth rate is very rapid. During the first year of life a baby should have per pound of body weight per day
   1. 0.5 grams protein.
   2. 1.5 grams protein.
   3. 3.0 grams protein

313

5. There is disagreement about the merits of certain popular foods. Some people approve of the traditional "hot dog" at ball parks and amusement parks, but look askance at them when they're served to the small fry when the family is out for Sunday dinner. What is your opinion of the nutritional value of frankfurters and luncheon meats? Which of the following statements is true?

   a. They are made of inferior meats and therefore have lower-quality proteins than most meats.
   b. Although it does not have as much protein as most lean meats, one frankfurter furnishes as much protein as one ounce of cheese.
   c. They are a concentrated form of protein and therefore are much richer in protein than most meats.

6. The recommended daily allowance for iron for an adult is ten milligrams for a man and eighteen milligrams for a woman. Meat is one of our important sources of iron. How would you rank the following?

   a. Four ounces of roast beef.
   b. Four ounces of salami.
   c. Four ounces of chicken.
   d. Four ounces of liverwurst.

7. Sulfur—a tonic or a dangerous "additive"? The old-time remedy of sulfur and molasses—did it have any virtue? And what about dried fruits treated with sulfur? Proponents of so-called "natural" foods decry this as bad. Actually, sulfur is found in hundreds of compounds. It is a component of animal and vegetable tissue and has countless industrial uses. But what of its nutritional properties? Mark the following statements *true* (T) or *false* (F).

   a. Sulfur is an essential element present in all body cells and in many of the body fluids and hormones.
   b. The sulfur dioxide used in processing dried fruits is a source of excessive amounts of sulfur in the human diet.
   c. Foods containing sulfur need to be emphasized in the diet since so much is lost through the growth of hair and nails.
   d. The requirement for sulfur in human beings has not yet been established, but it is probably related to protein requirements.

8. Most of us learned as children that calcium in milk is needed for strong bones and teeth and that we get vitamin C from orange juice. But how much do you really know about food? Answer these questions and see.

   A. Which of the following foods has the most calcium?
      1. A one-inch cube (one ounce) of cheddar cheese.
      2. Three ounces of sardines.
      3. An eight-ounce glass of milk.
   B. If you wanted to get the most vitamin C, what would you choose?
      1. One cup cooked broccoli.
      2. One medium orange.
      3. One medium tomato.

9. Approximately one hundred substances, some with strange-sounding scientific names, have been identified in our foods. Most of us know about proteins, minerals such as calcium and iron, and the alphabet of vitamins, but very few know all about all. How many are you familiar with? For example, what is inositol?
  - a. It is one of the B-complex vitamins.
  - b. It is an essential fatty acid found in peanut oil.
  - c. It, along with ergosterol, is a form of vitamin D.

10. Everyone is talking about fats. Some proclaim that there are "good fats" and "bad fats." Others maintain that "polyunsaturates" can rejuvenate man and invigorate his best friend, the dog. What do you know about fats?
  - a. Is it true or is it false that fats are a good food?
  - b. Is it true or is it false that vegetable oils are lower in calories than animal fats?
  - c. Is it true or is it false that "polyunsaturates" are some kind of magic fat?
  - d. Is it true or is it false that "polyunsaturates" are beneficial in the prevention of heart disease?
  - e. Is it true or is it false that low-fat diets are good?

11. If you are watching your waistline and counting calories, which of these foods would add the fewest calories to your salad?
  - a. One tablespoon sour cream.
  - b. One tablespoon mayonnaise.
  - c. One tablespoon salad oil such as Wesson or Mazola.

12. Most people regard beverages as refreshments, not food. However, some beverages, such as milk, are important sources of nutrients. Does beer have any unusual nutritional value? Which of the following statements about beer do you think is true?
  - a. Beer is one of our richest sources of riboflavin, due to its malt content.
  - b. Beer is advocated by some as an aid to those who are underweight.
  - c. Beer is a liquid beverage that supplies calories and trace amounts of minerals and vitamins.

13. Ice cream is probably one of our few really "national" dishes. It is common—it is ubiquitous—but what do you know about it as far as its contribution to our nutrition is concerned? How many calories are there in one-half pint (one cup) of the following?

  A. Vanilla ice cream:
  1. 100 calories.
  2. 200 calories.
  3. 300 calories.

  B. Lemon sherbet:
  1. 75 calories.
  2. 150 calories.
  3. 235 calories.

  C. Frozen custard or ice milk:
  1. 200 calories.
  2. 285 calories.
  3. 325 calories.

14. We are sure you have heard a lot about "royal jelly." Do you know what it is? See if you can choose the right answer from the three statements below.

        a. It is a preserve made from a tropical fruit.

        b. It is the food of the queen bee, a substance from the salivary glands of the worker bees.

        c. It is a gelatin dessert.

15. Everyone has heard of wheat germ, but do you know what it is? Can you pick the correct answer?

        a. It is a bacteria that causes a disease of the wheat plant.

        b. It is the portion of the wheat kernel called the embryo, from which the new plant starts its growth.

        c. It is the vitamin-rich outer covering of the wheat kernel.

16. Is honey better for you than "regular" sugar? Should one use the unpurified forms of sugar such as molasses and sorghum? Test your knowledge about these foods. Are these statements true or false?

        a. Honey can be used by diabetics as a substitute for table sugar since it is a "natural" sugar and therefore not harmful.

        b. Molasses is a better health builder than refined sugar because it supplies more energy and is a good source of other essential nutrients.

        c. The sugar sorbitol can be used freely in place of regular sugar because it is not utilized by the body.

ANSWERS

1. This question is typical of the confusion created in most of our minds by the nutrition discussions we hear and read. There is no unqualified answer. According to all the surveys and diet studies on individuals, groups, and families, as well as from the information compiled by the United States Department of Agriculture from "food disappearance" figures, the people of the United States are more adequately nourished *as a population* than any other people in the world and at any other time in history.

In the 1930s it was estimated that approximately one-third of American families were poorly fed. At the present time only 10 percent of families have diets below the standard used in the thirties. We don't need to feel smug, however. It is believed that this 10 percent is ill-fed as much because of lack of knowledge as from poverty. Also, 10 percent is a large number—several million families. It behooves us all to make every effort to correct even this "small amount."

By looking at the insurance actuarial figures with respect to weight it appears that a sizable segment of the American population is overnourished, at least as far as calories are concerned. Therefore, a, b, c, and d are all correct to a degree, depending on one's point of view.

2. Pasteurization does not affect the nutrients we depend upon milk to provide—principally protein, riboflavin, calcium, and vitamin A. The process does reduce the ascorbic acid and, to a lesser degree, the thiamine (vitamin B_1) content of milk. But, remember, milk is a poor source of these two nutrients anyway and also of iron.

   Pasteurization decreases the bacterial content of the milk, destroying the pathogens (disease-producing bacteria), thus increasing the value of milk as a safe, wholesome food.

3. The nutritive qualities of canned evaporated milk are every bit as good as those of fresh pasteurized milk. It has the added advantage of being homogenized, of having vitamin D added, of being inexpensive and absolutely clean. Some people consider its flavor as being inferior to fresh milk; others think it superior.

4. A. (3) is correct. At five or six months of age the infant may need 55 to 60 Calories per pound if particularly active. Both human and cow's milk supply about 21 Calories per ounce.

   B. (2) is correct. If the mother's iron intake has been adequate, babies have a high hemoglobin level at birth. By about three months of age the level has gone down to a fairly normal figure. At this time some iron-containing foods such as egg yolk, green vegetables, and cereals may be added. It does very little good to give dietary iron earlier. Milk, both human and cow's, is low in iron.

   C. Again (2) is the right answer. There is no clear indication that as long as part of the protein is from a good source, such as milk, meat, or egg, that any more than 1.5 grams is needed by the young baby. Human milk supplies about 0.36 grams per ounce. Cow's milk has more—about 1 gram per ounce.

5. Both (a) and (c) are false; (b) is true. Contrary to opinions held by some people, frankfurters and luncheon meats are good food and furnish high-quality protein.

6. I'm sure you all know that liver is rich in iron, but how many of you placed liverwurst first in this list? The correct order is (d), (a) and (b) are tied, and (c) comes last. Four ounces of liverwurst has six milligrams of iron, the roast beef and salami have four, and the chicken has a little more than two milligrams. But this does not mean that all these foods are not good sources of this important nutrient. Even though as a meat chicken is relatively low in iron, the frequency with which it is used can make it a fairly substantial source of this nutrient.

7. The correct answers are (a) true, (b) false, (c) false, and (d) true. And to elaborate (a), since sulfur is a component of most proteins, thus accounting for most of the sulfur in the body, it can be considered an essential nutrient. It is found in some enzymes, two known vitamins as well as insulin. Hair contains 4 to 6 percent sulfur.

(b) For human beings, it appears that inorganic forms of sulfur are not available to the body. In processing some dried fruits the inorganic compound sulfur dioxide is used as an antioxidant to prevent and to protect somewhat against a loss of vitamin C and vitamin A activity. It does destroy some thiamine, but fruits are not good sources of this vitamin, while they are of vitamins C and A.

(c) Very little is known about the use of sulfur in the human body. A few studies on hair growth and wool production have given no evidence of any relationship between these and an excess or deficiency in intake of sulfur-containing amino acids.

(d) Although this is true, it is known that protein foods supply the major amount. It may be possible for the body to utilize the simple organic forms found in some other foods such as onions, cabbage, beans, nuts.

Therefore, as far as our present knowledge is concerned, sulfur is essential to human nutrition, but is evidently abundantly supplied.

8. A. You'll probably be surprised to know that (2) is the correct answer. Sardines owe their high calcium content to their tiny, edible bones. Three ounces of sardines have 328 milligrams of calcium, the milk, 288 milligrams, and the cheese, 206 milligrams.

    B. Here again, the correct answer will come as a surprise to you—(a) is the right answer. One cup of cooked broccoli contains 110 milligrams of vitamin C, a medium orange, 75 milligrams, and the tomato has 35 milligrams of vitamin C. But, in reality, all three of these foods are good sources of this vitamin, and we ought to have at least 50 to 75 milligrams of vitamin C each day.

9. The correct answer is (a). Inositol has been shown to be required for growth and health in experimental animals, but its role in human nutrition is not yet known. Heart, liver, wheat germ, yeast, and whole-grain cereals are known as good food sources of this vitamin.

10. (a) Fats are certainly good; in fact, no one can live without fat. Why? (1) Fats are a fine concentrated source of the fuel that the body requires for the functioning of its life processes. (2) Fats carry vitamins and fatty acids essential for health. (3) Fats, when stored in the body in moderate amounts, provide an energy reserve, a padding for vital organs, and insulation against extremes of temperature. (4) Fats give flavor to a meal and add "staying power" because they slow down the rate at which food is digested.

    (b) This is false. In calorie value, all edible fats are alike. Vegetable oils come from corn, cottonseeds, olives, soybeans, and nuts. Animal fat is in beef, pork, lamb, poultry, fish, and in milk. Whatever the source, every teaspoon of fat supplies about forty Calories of energy. Fats differ, though, in other ways; so a varied food intake is necessary to insure a good balance of all the fats.

(c) This is false. A fat is saturated or unsaturated just as a person is tall or short. All fats contain a substance called glycerol and also one or more fatty acids. These fatty acids differ from each other in their content of elements known as hydrogen and carbon. Fats that are liquid or soft at room temperature contain fatty acids with less hydrogen and are known as unsaturated. If they are very short of hydrogen, they are called polyunsaturated. Hydrogenation can change an unsaturated oil into a solid, saturated fat, but light hydrogenation makes only a little saturated fat.

(d) No one knows. Some studies indicate that in countries where people use large amounts of vegetable oils (as in southern Italy), they tend to have low blood cholesterol levels and a low death rate from heart disease. Such observations have created the current interest in vegetable oils and in the margarines that contain a high proportion of unsaturated fatty acids. However, much is still puzzling. Positive conclusions must await the results of further research.

(e) The amount of fat that is good depends on an individual's need. If you are in good health, and if you are maintaining weight your doctor says is good for you, the chances are that you are not eating too much fat. Unfortunately, though, in the United States, millions of people are overweight, and eating too much, including too much fat. For these, it is important to cut down on most food and drink, including fats. Moderation and consumption of a variety of all kinds of foods assure the amount of fat, and of minerals, proteins, vitamins, and other essentials, that are desirable for desirable weight and for good health.

11. Sour-cream lovers will be glad to know that (a) is the right answer. Tablespoon for tablespoon, it has about one-third as many calories as mayonnaise and one-fourth as many calories as salad oil. One tablespoon of sour cream would add 30 Calories to your salad, while the mayonnaise has 90 Calories and the salad oil about 125 Calories.

12. Both (b) and (c) are correct, because beer is chiefly a source of calories. An eight-ounce glass of beer has about 112 Calories. It has only a trace of thiamine, riboflavin, and iron, but provides reasonable amounts of one of the B-vitamins called niacin.

13. The answers are (3), (3), and (2). Regular ice cream has the most calories. Actually, there is more of a difference than these figures show, for if they were based on weight rather than volume, ice cream would be considerably higher since it weighs less for any given volume than sherbet or ice milk. There is more air incorporated into it.

14. The right answer is (b). Although you may have heard rumors, royal jelly doesn't preserve anything but the queen bee. Ladies, don't count too heavily on its preservative powers as far as your complexion is concerned. It's worth a king's ransom, however. A price we've seen quoted is $140 an ounce—gold goes for about the same!

15. You're right if you chose (b). Wheat germ makes up about 2 to 5 percent of the weight of the wheat kernel and is a concentrated source of protein, iron, vitamin E, and the B vitamins.

16. The answers to all three of these are false. Honey is sugar in a liquid form rather than granular. It is about 20 percent water and 75 percent carbohydrate. There is no evidence that body cells differentiate between a molecule of glucose (blood sugar) that originated from honey and a molecule of glucose from any other source. Honey has no special virtues other than a taste and texture that many enjoy.

Again, molasses is an unrefined form of sugar. It does contain a higher amount of iron, calcium, and phosphorus than white sugar. But when one eats a varied diet the very small amounts of these minerals that might have come from molasses would make little difference to one's total nutrient intake. As for furnishing more energy than white sugar—NO—one tablespoon of each supplies almost the same number of calories.

Sorbitol is the alcohol derivative of a sugar called sorbose that is made from dextrose or corn sugar. It is absorbed very slowly from the intestinal tract, therefore makes little impression on the blood sugar level, but it is absorbed—and does contribute calories. Therefore, it must be accounted for—especially since for most people, the calorie content of the diet is as important as the carbohydrate content.